# CONTROLLING HEALTH
PROFESSIONALS

# STATE OF HEALTH SERIES

Edited by Chris Ham, Director of the Health Services Management Centre, University of Birmingham

*Current and forthcoming titles*

*Financing Health Care in the 1990s*
John Appleby

*Patients, Policies and Politics*
John Butler

*Going Private: Why People Pay For Their Health Care*
Michael Calnan, Sarah Cant and Jonathan Gabe

*Controlling Health Professionals*
Stephen Harrison and Christopher Pollitt

*Public Law and Health Service Accountability*
Diane Longley

*Hospitals in Transition*
Tim Packwood, Justin Keen and Martin Buxton

*Planned Markets and Public Competition*
Richard B. Saltman and Casten von Otter

*Whose Standards? Consumer and Professional Standards in Health Care*
Charlotte Williamson

# CONTROLLING HEALTH PROFESSIONALS

The Future of Work and Organization in the National Health Service

## Stephen Harrison and Christopher Pollitt

**Open University Press**
Buckingham · Philadelphia

Open University Press
Celtic Court
22 Ballmoor
Buckingham
MK18 1XW

and
1900 Frost Road, Suite 101
Bristol, PA 19007, USA

First Published 1994

A catalogue record of this book is available from the British Library

ISBN 0–335–09643–3 (pbk)    0–335–09644–1 (hbk)

**Library of Congress Cataloging-in-Publication Data**

Harrison, Stephen, 1947–
    Controlling health professionals: the future of work and organization
in the National Health Service/Stephen Harrison and Christopher
Pollitt.
        p.    cm. – (State of health series)
    Includes bibliographical references and index.
    ISBN 0–335–09644–1 (hbk)    ISBN 0–335–09643–3 (pbk)
    1. National Health Service (Great Britain) – Personnel
management.    2. National Health Service (Great Britain) –
Administration.    3. Medical personnel – Government policy – Great
Britain.
I. Pollitt, Christopher.    II. Title.    III. Series.
RA412.5.G7H33    1994                                                    93–2325
362.1′068 – dc20                                                            CIP

Typeset by Type Study, Scarborough
Printed in Great Britain by St Edmundsbury Press,
Bury St Edmunds, Suffolk

# CONTENTS

# SERIES EDITOR'S INTRODUCTION

Health services in many developed countries have come under critical scrutiny in recent years. In part this is because of increasing expenditure, much of it funded from public sources, and the pressure this has put on governments seeking to control public spending. Also important has been the perception that resources allocated to health services are not always deployed in an optimal fashion. Thus at a time when the scope for increasing expenditure is extremely limited, there is a need to search for ways of using existing budgets more efficiently. A further concern has been the desire to ensure access to health care of various groups on an equitable basis. In some countries this has been linked to a wish to enhance patient choice and to make service providers more responsive to patients as 'consumers'.

Underlying these specific concerns are a number of more fundamental developments which have a significant bearing on the performance of health services. Three are worth highlighting. First, there are demographic changes, including the ageing population and the decline in the proportion of the population of working age. These changes will both increase the demand for health care and at the same time limit the ability of health services to respond to this demand.

Second, advances in medical science will also give rise to new demands within the health services. These advances cover a range of possibilities, including innovations in surgery, drug therapy, screening and diagnosis. The pace of innovation is likely to quicken as the end of the century approaches, with significant implications for the funding and provision of services.

Third, public expectations of health services are rising as those who use services demand higher standards of care. In part, this is stimulated by developments within the health service, including the availability of new technology. More fundamentally, it stems from the emergence of a more educated and informed population, in which people are accustomed to being treated as consumers rather than patients.

Against this background, policy makers in a number of countries are reviewing the future of health services. Those countries which have traditionally relied on a market in health care are making greater use of regulation and planning. Equally, those countries which have traditionally relied on regulation and planning are moving towards a more competitive approach. In no country is there complete satisfaction with existing methods of financing and delivery, and everywhere there is a search for new policy instruments.

The aim of this series is to contribute to debate about the future of health services through an analysis of major issues in health policy. These issues have been chosen because they are both of current interest and of enduring importance. The series is intended to be accessible to students and informed lay readers as well as to specialists working in this field. The aim is to go beyond a textbook approach to health policy analysis and to encourage authors to move debate about their issue forward. In this sense, each book presents a summary of current research and thinking, and an exploration of future policy directions.

Professor Chris Ham
Director of the Health Services Management Centre,
University of Birmingham

# GLOSSARY OF ABBREVIATIONS

BMA      British Medical Association
CEPOD    Confidential Enquiry into Perioperative Deaths
CHC      Community Health Council
DGM      District General Manager
DHA      District Health Authority
DHSS     Department of Health and Social Security
DMU      Directly Managed Unit
DOH      Department of Health
DRG      Diagnosis-Related Group
GDP      Gross Domestic Product
GP       General [Medical] Practitioner
HCHS     Hospital and Community Health Services
MB       Management Budget
NHS      National Health Service
NVQ      National Vocational Qualification
PAC      Committee of Public Accounts
PRO      Professional Review Organization
PSBR     Public Sector Borrowing Requirement
RCN      Royal College of Nursing
RGM      Regional General Manager
RHA      Regional Health Authority
RM       Resource Management
TQM      Total Quality Management
UGM      Unit General Manager
UKCC     United Kingdom Central Council for Nursing, Mid-
         wifery and Health Visiting

# INTRODUCTION

This book is one of a series concerned with the future of the UK's National Health Service (NHS). In this volume, we are concerned with work and organization; as the title suggests, we see the key issue as being the means by which professional work will be controlled.

In Chapter 1, we explain what we mean by 'professional' and why we have placed professional workers at the centre of our analysis. We also provide an account of the 'backdrop': changes in the public sector in general, of which the subject matter of our book is just a part. In Chapter 2, we present the theoretical basis of our analysis, since we cannot discuss the future without some (implicit or explicit) notion about how the world 'works'. We prefer to be as explicit as the space available in this short book allows. In Chapter 2, and throughout the book, we have dealt with theories by explaining their content, rather than labelling them by author or *genre*. Readers who wish to investigate further will find appropriate references at the end of each chapter.

Chapters 3, 4 and 5 each explore one broad approach to controlling professionals, examining recent developments and making some assessment of prospects for the immediate future. There is a degree of overlap, both logical and chronological, between these. Chapter 3 is concerned with traditional managerial control: attacking the professions directly. In this category we include the development of general management and performance indicators, and also an account of some challenges to professional associations and trade unions. Chapter 4 is concerned with what we term the 'incorporation' of professionals into management. By this, we mean strategies for controlling professionals indirectly, by subtlely changing their attitudes and perceptions, and thereby changing what is sometimes called the 'culture' of the organization. Included here are decentralized budgeting and resource management, the development of forms of organization involving 'clinical directorates', and the spread of professionally-based forms of evaluation, such as medical audit. In Chapter 5, we consider approaches to controlling the professions which consist in changing the larger environment in which the NHS operates. These include the institutionalized split of 'purchaser' and 'provider' roles, and the ostensible empowerment of health care consumers.

Chapter 6 contains our conclusions: although much of our analysis so far suggests that managers have achieved an increasing degree of control over health professionals, we do not see this as a process with a long-term future. Rather, we believe, the future of professional health work lies increasingly in independent clinical practice, though, of course, also in management itself.

The overall purpose of this book (as of the series of which it forms part) is to stimulate debate and discussion. We have chosen to focus on the macro-pressures which we believe to be shaping the environment in which the health professions operate, rather than by attempting any prescriptions of our own. Nevertheless, it would be absurd to pretend that none of our own value-judgements lurk beneath our analysis. Briefly, we acknowledge the genuine concern and dedication of health professionals and empathize with their discomfort at being asked to operate in ways very different from the assumptions that led them to their career choices. (As university academics we suffer parallel discomforts.) At the same time we sympathize with NHS managers caught between professionals and government. But we also share a more-than-healthy scepticism about the other motives of both groups; in recent years the occupational advancement activities of managers have often been as self-interested as those of professionals over a longer period.

Although we believe our book is soundly based in academic work, it is intended for general readership. We have decided, therefore to keep references to a minimum. Inevitably, we will have failed to properly acknowledge all our intellectual debts, and we unreservedly apologize to our creditors.

We wish, however, to take this opportunity to acknowledge the various forms of support in the preparation of this book provided by

Chris Ham (our series editor), Rockwell Schulz (who provided the idyllic location in which Chapter 1 was written), Charlotte Armour (who typed the manuscript), Andrew Green (who checked our economics), Colin Thunhurst (who provided the calculations incorporated into our assessment of the adequacy of NHS resource growth – see Figure 2.4) and to Richard Baggaley, formerly of the Open University Press, for his forbearance in the face of our constant rescheduling of the manuscript. We remain, of course, responsible for the final text.

# PROFESSIONALS AND MANAGERS

In this chapter we set the scene for what follows. There are two main sections. The first offers an analysis of the character of professionalism itself and explores some reasons why certain aspects of professionalism pose problems for those charged with running public service organizations such as the UK National Health Service (NHS). The second section then describes the broad backdrop against which the particular developments within the NHS need to be understood. Whilst the NHS has – as subsequent chapters will show – many peculiarities, it would be a mistake to think that what has happened to managers and professionals has been unique or unconnected to wider developments in the UK public services sector as a whole.

## PROFESSIONALS

Professionals are not, of course, the only NHS workers, nor the only ones to have been the objects of managerial attention in recent years. Indeed, some of the developments in the management of professionals which we shall examine in later chapters rely upon concepts and experience derived from earlier strategies (such as competitive tendering) for managing non-professional staff. More than half of NHS staff, however, consider themselves to be professionals; we are concerned in this book with the future of perhaps half a million people.

More importantly, professionals present a crucial problem for management because of the close association between professional-ism and autonomy. Broadly speaking, there are three different notions of professionalism in welfare state organizations such as the NHS, all of which encompass some notion of autonomy. If (to put it rather crudely) professionalism involves acting on autonomous judgement, and management involves getting other people to do what one wants, then there is a potential conflict. It is important to note that such conflict does not *necessarily* occur; as we show in the second part of this chapter, the history of the NHS from 1948 to the early 1980s exhibits very little of it, at least in overt form. The conflict *will* occur (as indeed has been the case) when managers press professionals to behave in ways which the latter do not want. Chapter 2 examines why this has happened.[1]

The first of our three notions of professionalism stresses the functionality of professional arrangements for clients and patients. Roughly speaking, the argument goes as follows. Being the client or patient of a professional is different from being the customer in a normal exchange relationship; the patient lacks knowledge of the health problem and of what might appropriately be done about it. Consequently, to enter into a relationship with a professional means entrusting one's interests to that professional. In order to provide conditions in which such trust is not exploited, two pro-fessional freedoms are necessary. One is that the professional must be free from outside interference in exercising his or her expert knowledge in the interests of the patient. The other is that the profession as a body must be largely self-regulating; patients need to be protected from charlatans and incompetent practitioners, but only the profession itself can provide such protection since only it possesses the necessary technical knowledge. It is this view of professionalism which is most often deployed by the professions themselves either because it most closely fits the self-image ac-quired during training and practice and/or because it allows them to occupy moral high ground.

Our second notion of professionalism is a stark contrast – a strategy by which groups of workers pursue 'occupational control', that is, more congenial conditions of work for themselves. Essen-tially, it is argued, professionals employ the rhetoric of the first notion set out above, but actually act in pursuit of self-interest rather than client/patient interest. Thus the characteristics of pro-fessionalism such as autonomy and self-regulation help to produce a situation in which managerial control and supervision can be evaded, and in which the practice of specific skills can be retained as a monopoly within the profession, helping to keep earnings higher, and career prospects better, than would otherwise have been the case.

The third notion of professionalism is different again. The argument is roughly as follows. The autonomy enjoyed by professionals is partly illusory; their judgements are, in fact, heavily influenced by the socialization that they have received during training. This socialization is oriented towards the perception of illness as an individual pathology rather than one which is socially, politically or economically created. Such a view or ideology is non-threatening to the state because it places the causes of illness either in biological contingencies for which no-one can be held responsible, or in individual lifestyles for which the victim can be blamed. Nevertheless, professionals are left with just enough operating autonomy for the state to be able to evade the politically awkward decisions about how to ration the finite resources available for health services. (We examine the issue of rationing in more detail in Chapter 2.) Because these rationing decisions are highly fragmented into individual transactions between patients and professionals, they are politically invisible. There are no statistics about the number of patients denied treatment or about the 'corners cut' in the care provided to them. Representatives of the government may, however, defend these arrangements in the rhetoric of the first notion.

We have stressed how very different from each other are these notions. This does not mean, however, that they are contradictory. Our view is that they all reflect aspects of reality. Professionalism is all three things, and there is something in it to suit both patients, professionals, and the state. This is why it will be necessary to spend some time, in Chapter 2, explaining why anyone should want to upset this *status quo*.

It may now be helpful to flesh out the three abstract notions of professionalism by providing some illustrations about how they apply to the NHS. We begin by looking at the medical profession, often employed as the archetype for this type of analysis.

Our first notion is illustrated by all the paraphernalia of state registration. In the case of medicine, the Medical Act forbids non-qualified persons to represent themselves as registered practitioners; the General Medical Council (the majority of whose members are doctors) recognizes qualifications and registers suitably qualified persons. The Council also carries out a disciplinary function, and may 'strike off' practitioners who breach its code of conduct. These arrangements are formally created by government, and have, since the creation of the NHS, been buttressed by government commitment to the notion of 'clinical freedom'. This concept is nowhere formally defined, though is generally taken to constitute something like the right of a fully-qualified doctor to diagnose and treat his or her patients as he or she wishes, within the limits of available resources. As recently as December 1979, the Conservative Government consultation document *Patients First* (DHSS and Welsh Office 1979) noted:

> It is doctors, dentists and nurses and their colleagues in the other health professions who provide the care and cure of patients and promote the health of the people. It is the purpose of management to support them in giving that service.

In addition, the self-regulatory character of medicine is enhanced by the role of the Royal Colleges and Faculties in determining the character and content of medical specialization.

Our second notion of professionalism – occupational control – is evident in several aspects of medicine. First, doctors frequently use the principle of clinical freedom to extend their control beyond the strictly clinical and into issues of resource allocation (such as quasi-ownership of hospital beds) and working practices more generally. Second, doctors have largely been able to arrange their work to suit their own clinical and intellectual preferences; there is a real sense in which the overall shape of health services provided in the UK has been largely the aggregate of individual clinical decisions, for instance (in the 1970s) to use additional financial resources to diagnose and treat patients more intensively rather than to treat more patients. Third, the collegial character of the profession, in which all fully qualified practitioners (specialists and GPs) are treated as peers, rather than as working in hierarchical relationships, militates very much against the ability of outsiders to gain control. (We examine the implications of clinical directorates in Chapter 4.) Fourth, the medical profession buttresses its own position through widespread involvement in the training and state registration of other health professions as well as itself, based on a widely accepted claim that medical knowledge is all-encompassing of health services, other professions therefore being logically subordinate.

Our third notion of professionalism is manifest in the very clear individually-oriented model of ill health (sometimes referred to as the 'medical model') upon which the NHS is constructed despite the plentiful evidence of the relatively greater importance of other factors in causing ill health. Functions such as health promotion and disease prevention have been treated as marginal and low in status, whilst most occupational and environmental health are outside the service altogether. Moreover, it is equally clear that clinical decisions about treatment constitute a hidden process of rationing which government would rather not be involved in; it is difficult to imagine a Cabinet Minister, for instance, seeing anything but political *disadvantage* in becoming involved in decisions about the allocation to patients of scarce places for (say) renal dialysis. Yet renal physicians make such decisions almost as a matter of routine.

We mentioned above that medicine is frequently cited as the archetypal profession, and it will already be evident that the other health professions are not precisely analogous. We mentioned, for instance, medical involvement in the training and state registration of other groups. There are close similarities, however; almost the whole of the patient-oriented notion of professionalism can be applied to the other clinical professions. Much of the third notion also applies, though perhaps less dramatically than in the case of medicine. Nurses and physiotherapists, for instance, may well be involved in deciding the frequency of visits, respectively, to a domiciliary patient or by a rehabilitation patient.

Although some non-medical professions (such as dentistry and midwifery) do exhibit considerable degrees of independent practice, and other professions (such as physiotherapy) have from time to time been involved in conflicts over their autonomy from the medical profession, their major divergence from the three notions of professional autonomy is in the area of occupational control. Whilst some aspects of this (influence over 'manpower' planning, for instance) parallel medicine, others do not. Most importantly, the occupational control strategies of the other professions have not rested upon collegial arrangements. Instead, there have been, since the mid-1960s, three related elements.

First, the non-medical professions have been able to construct managerial hierarchies exclusive to themselves. This has both ensured that professionals were not managed by persons from outside the particular profession and guaranteed promotion opportunities for members of the profession. Thus, the Salmon Report of 1966 took it as axiomatic that nurses' status was too low and made recommendations (which were implemented, and survived more or less intact until 1984) for an extensive nurse managerial hierarchy in hospitals. Though not on the same scale, similar arrangements were developed for community nursing (the Mayston Report), scientists and technicians (the Zuckerman Report), pharmacists (the Noel Hall Report) and physiotherapists, occupational therapists, radiographers, remedial gymnasts, dietitians, chiropodists, orthoptists and speech therapists (the Halsbury Report). This trend reached its apogee in 1974 in the organization structure of the reorganized NHS. The top managers of nursing were members of consensus management teams, equal in status to chief administrators, whilst the top managers in other professions, although not members of the consensus team itself, reported to the team rather than to an individual outside their own profession. (We discuss these teams in more detail below.) Despite occasional ostensible attempts to reward clinical responsibility (such as in the clinical grading structures of the late 1980s), the career prospects of the non-medical professions lie mainly within management.

Second, some of the non-medical professions have succeeded in creating a series of residual, largely unskilled, occupations to take over the less-interesting 'non-professional' aspects of their work, whilst remaining firmly under professional control. Nursing auxiliaries/assistants, and physiotherapy and occupational therapy aides/helpers, are examples of such occupations. Conflict has occasionally occurred over such groups: between nurses and domestic services managers in the late 1970s over control of ward orderlies and domestic assistants, for instance. As we shall see in Chapter 3, it is possible for the growth of such groups to threaten the professions.

Third, at least one occupation, nursing, has consciously been developing its clinical base, potentially in opposition to medicine. The 'new nursing' is based on the notion that nursing work is therapeutic in its own right, rather than simply 'maintenance work' for doctors.[2]

Summarizing the first section of this chapter, then, we can say that health professionals constitute a potential problem for management, either because (as in medicine) of their claim to non-managed status or because (as in most of the other professions) of their claim to be managed exclusively by members of their own profession.

## THE BACKDROP: THE RESTRUCTURING OF THE
## UK PUBLIC SERVICES SECTOR

Few working in the public services can have failed to notice that the way in which they are organized and managed has been in a state of upheaval since the late 1970s, and especially since the late 1980s. On the whole, this change process has been driven by central government and on the whole the public service professions have been perceived by the Government as obstacles to rather than allies in the business of reform.

The original impulse for reform was not simple, and embraced a variety of economic and ideological components. Economically, the British Government, in common with almost all its counterparts in western Europe, read the lessons of the great mid-1970s bout of stagflation as meaning that rates of growth in aggregate public expenditure must be curbed.[3] Even before the advent of Mrs Thatcher's administration in 1979 the Labour Government had made sharp cuts in public service spending. The welfare state could hardly hope to escape the new restraints since it was the most rapidly growing element of public expenditure during the early and mid-1970s. Three of the four largest spending programmes were of this type – health care, education and, by far the largest of all, social security (defence was the fourth big spender). The detailed financial arithmetic concerning the NHS will be explored further in the next chapter.

Ideologically, the 1979 General Election brought to power an increasingly radical right-wing Conservative administration, led by a Prime Minister whose personal suspicions of self-interested behaviour by public service staff were well known. The 'New Right' or neo-liberal wing of the Conservatives held to a body of theoretical beliefs which portrayed public services as inefficient, costly monopolies which used their influence over information to ensure that more services were provided than the average voter wanted to afford.[4] Within this unflattering portrait the public service professions were singled out for particular criticism. Set in their ways, it was suggested that such professionals used their job security (greater than the private sector could afford) as a basis for empire building and resistance to those who wished to reform them. From their entrenched professional strongholds they were also able to ensure that the *content* of the services they provided was shaped by their own predilections more than by what governments or the

citizens using these services might actually want. This was, therefore, a fairly virulent version of the *occupational control* notion of
professionalism – professions acted in their own selfish interests and
in 'restraint of trade'.

Perhaps the first major assault on the professional strongholds
began when Mrs Thatcher's Labour predecessor, James Callaghan,
invaded the schoolteachers' 'secret garden' of the curriculum. In a
major speech in 1976 he declared that:

> 'To the teachers I would say that you must satisfy the parents
> and industry that what you are doing meets the requirements
> and needs of their children.'

Criticisms of professional unresponsiveness, long-standing currency on the political left, were appropriated and enlarged by the
New Right. For Mrs Thatcher and her co-believers, however, the
solution to the problem was very different from that previously
envisaged by the left. Where the left of the late 1960s and early
1970s had espoused *participation* by the users of public services, the
New Right turned to the private sector and sought better *management*. Better management would come through the catalyst of
privatization and exposure to the competitive forces of the market
or, where that was not practicable, by introducing to the residual
public sector, private-sector models of dynamic general management. Such managers would ensure that professional restrictive
practices were progressively eliminated and that individual professionals were obliged to fall more closely in line with overall
organizational objectives.

The first wave of Thatcherite managerialism ran from 1979 until
the mid-1980s. It comprised a determined drive to impose greater
economy and efficiency. Cost-consciousness, 'savings' and the dissemination of the skills of financial management were the leading
characteristics of changes introduced in many public services.
'Rayner scrutinies' were brought into play, first in the civil service
and later in the NHS. From 1982 all Whitehall departments had to
offer up contributions to the Financial Management Initiative
(FMI). In the NHS 'cost improvement programmes' became a
feature of daily life, and the emphasis of the planning process
turned from longer-term strategy towards tightly costed short-term
operational plans. Central government introduced the first national
set of NHS performance indicators (from 1983) and encouraged
health authorities to experiment with management budgeting. The

NHS was far from being alone in all this. Apart from similar innovations in the civil service performance indicators (mainly measuring economy and efficiency) were developed for local education authorities and other local government services, the police and the universities. In almost all parts of the public service sector considerable investments were made in computerized management information systems and these frequently gave salience to specifically financial information.

By the mid to late 1980s, the limitations of this 'economy and efficiency' strategy were beginning to become apparent to ministers and their advisers. In brief, it was a strategy with only limited appeal to either the staff of the public services themselves or, more importantly perhaps, the electorate. There was evidence of widespread demoralization of both teachers and NHS staff who experienced 'economy and efficiency' as a series of cuts, and who not infrequently perceived the Government as being 'against them'. This latter view was perhaps understandable in the light of the Government's willingness to 'take on' the public service unions during major strike actions, and a steady trickle of disparaging remarks from the New Right think tanks and, on occasion, ministers themselves. More fundamentally, the Government embarked on a series of industrial relations Acts which progressively restricted the freedoms hitherto enjoyed by trade unions.

The point here is not that public service professionals were indifferent to efforts to increase economy and efficiency. There can be little doubt that the early efforts of the Conservative administration yielded many worthwhile savings and enhanced the previously low levels of cost consciousness. Yet at the same time this was not a central or sufficient motivator for many public service staff. Improved efficiency, whilst gratifying, was not quite 'the point', and did not make up for the widespread belief that the public services were facing an ideologically unsympathetic and occasionally punitive regime. Most doctors, teachers, nurses and social workers had joined their professions with some notion, however vague, of 'doing good', but this vocational aspect (with its accompanying ethic of service improvement) seemed to find little echo on the Government side during the first half of the Thatcher decade.

However, it was probably *public* opinion which finally convinced ministers of the need to modify their approach. Surveys showed an increasing public disquiet at the state of the health and education services. Substantial majorities (even majorities of Conservative voters) began to say that they wanted to *increase* public expenditure, even if that meant a rise in their tax bills. Before both the 1987 and 1992 General Elections the Conservative leadership was fed poll information indicating that one of the areas in which Labour was more favourably regarded by the majority of the voters was that of the public services in general and the NHS in particular. Behind this there may well have been a deeper distrust of all political slogans and promises. Survey evidence tends to show that the British public reposes far greater trust in their doctors and teachers than in their elected representatives. So the endless parade of such professionals appearing in the media to bemoan the decline of these popular services is likely to have made more impact than ministerial rhetoric in favour of better management and the need for yet more savings.

Thus, from the late 1980s, a second wave of managerial reform began to wash over the UK public service sector. The original emphasis on economy and efficiency remained. But now there were also 'added ingredients', especially 'quality', cultural change and a major extension of market and market-like mechanisms. Let us take each of these in turn.

By the mid-1990s, the rhetoric of service 'quality' has become so prominent and pervasive that it is easy to forget how recent was the adoption of this particular vocabulary. Like so much else in the Conservative Government's repertoire it was borrowed from private sector management practice (and has been extensively 'sold' by private sector management consultants). Techniques such as Total Quality Management (TQM) and the application of the British quality standard BS5750 are direct imports from the business world. The emphasis on quality has been immense – and we will be examining its NHS manifestations in Chapter 4.[5] What is interesting is how many purposes this virtuous term can be made to serve. Most obviously it can be used to reassure a general public which is anxious about a perceived decline in their public services. Second, if skilfully presented, the drive for 'quality' might help to rescue the sagging morale of public service staff. This is particularly true of approaches like TQM which are built upon techniques for engaging the participation and commitment of as many staff as possible. Third, quality initiatives may provide opportunities for management to increase its knowledge of, and influence over, areas of professional discretion, not least because contemporary, management-style quality programmes frequently substitute explicit, management-formulated standards for what were previously implicit professional judgements of what was appropriate and adequate in a particular circumstance.

The concern with 'cultural change' is similarly multi-faceted. The basic idea is that the hearts and minds of public service staff need to be won over to a new attitude and style. But again it is noticeable that management is seen as the principal agent of change. Implicitly the old attitudes are inappropriate and need to be replaced. The new public service will be more responsive to its citizen users – quicker, friendlier, willing to provide more information in more digestible formats, easier to complain to when things go wrong. This is the spirit of Prime Minister Major's *Citizen's Charter* and of the 29 lesser charters to which, at the time of writing, it had given birth. It fits perfectly with the pursuit of quality and with the more general attempt by the Major administration to rehabilitate the Government's reputation as caring for the public services.

However, this is not the only face of charterism. Economy and efficiency have certainly not gone away, and neither has the Government's wish to shape and direct the autonomy of public service professionals. Thus the Treasury has secured agreement within Whitehall that the *Citizen's Charter* shall be 'resource neutral' (i.e. that it shall not lead overall to net additional expenditure) and it is clearly envisaged that the 'standards' which are central to the charter programme shall be set by management and worked to by all staff, including the professions. Management also leads the rush to consult users, and management decides how the resulting 'feedback' shall be used (or not used). There is a sense in which this represents a new ability for management to outflank the traditional claim of the professional that he or she is in touch with the client/patient and knows what they really need.

Probably the most fundamental feature of the 'second wave' has been the vast extension of market and market-like mechanisms into the heartlands of the public service sector. The NHS has been given its 'provider market' (see especially Chapter 5). Local government has been instructed to pursue the model of an 'enabling authority', no longer providing most services itself but purchasing them on a competitive basis from a variety of public, voluntary and commercial providers. Schools now have their own budgets (under the Local Management of Schools initiative) and compete for students. The funding arrangements for universities have been changed so that they, likewise, have to compete with each other, both for students and in the quality of their research. Their success in these two competitions determine what public funding they receive. From 1 April 1993 each local authority will have to publish extensive performance indicator data which will allow the public to compare their performance with those of all the other local authorities in England and Wales. Meanwhile, central government continues to search for possibilities for privatizing or putting out to competitive tender services which have previously been firmly within the directly-provided public sector. Targets for this process now include core professional services such as (in local government) architecture, engineering, library support, audit and inspection. This process was further accelerated by the November 1991 White Paper *Competing for Quality*.[6]

The unrelenting emphasis on the desirability of market or market-like mechanisms has considerable implications for professionals and managers alike. First, it implies a further move away from the traditional model of lifetime professional careers working under national terms and conditions of service. The public service providers of the future will be working within contract or contract-like agreements which will be time-limited and strictly costed. Central government is encouraging them to move towards a parallel model of employment: many of their staff (including some professionals) will be employed on term contracts, with well-specified work targets and standards and a growing performance-related element within their remuneration. This has already become common at top management levels and is set to spread.

Market-like competition also has an impact on what one might term 'professional solidarity'. Doctors or teachers or social workers working for one provider are potentially set against those working for rival providers (who might deprive them of their contracts). They must also be guarded in their dealings with professionals who work for purchasing/funding authorities. Skilful managers are able to use this argument to encourage staff to focus more closely on their standards and targets. More effort goes into both public relations (front of the shop) and cost control (back of the shop). Increasingly, professionals are expected to support the corporate image and to refrain from public criticism of their own institution.

In sum, therefore, there is now emerging a new vision of the public services sector of the future. Public services will be much less monolithic than in the 1960s and 1970s. Relatively small purchasing organizations will buy in services from a wide variety of providers, fostering competition between them wherever possible. Purchase will take place through contract or contract-like mechanisms which will specify the volume, type, quality and price of the services to be supplied. Purchasers will monitor the extent to which providers comply with these specifications (and providers will obviously need to monitor their own operations too). Central government will make and remake the broad rules and guidelines by which these public markets and quasi-markets will operate, and may be called upon to settle any major disputes between purchasers and providers. Within these new arrangements permanent careers on nationally-determined salary scales will become much less common. A higher proportion of staff (professional and otherwise) will be employed on fixed-term contracts with locally-determined terms and conditions.

Very broadly, the implications of this new vision for the theme of this book are that management authority will expand and professional autonomy diminish. Also, job security for virtually all occupational groups is likely to decline. Efficiency should further increase, as should responsiveness to service users. Decisions about service priorities and standards should become more transparent, visible both in contracts and in published provider standards.

But all this is to assume that the vision of the 'second wave' will actually come to pass. That is far from a foregone conclusion, either in the NHS or in any other public service. In the following chapters we will examine how the broad concerns of both the first and second waves of public service reform were translated into the specifics of change and pressures for change within the NHS. We will consider how change has manifested itself at the interface between the most powerful and influential groups of NHS staff, and what the chances are that the vision of *Working for Patients* and the *Patient's Charter* will be realized.

# FINANCE FOR HEALTH CARE: SUPPLY, DEMAND AND RATIONING

This chapter is divided into four main sections. In the first, we show some of the major pressures on the supply of government resources for the welfare state in general and the NHS in particular. In the second, we give an account of the major demands upon these resources. In the third, we discuss rationing, the necessary consequence of an excess of demand over supply. In particular, we argue that most of the managerial developments which have taken place in the NHS during the 1980s represent a new gloss on a rationing process which has existed since 1948. Finally, we look at the future prospects; the 1990s, we argue, are unlikely to make much of a break in this pattern; this is likely to be the future for health professionals.

Before we begin our analysis, however, a word about theory is appropriate. In this book we are concerned with (as our subtitle makes clear) the future of professional work in the NHS. In order to make forecasts about the future, we cannot avoid having a theory: a belief, or set of related beliefs, about how the world in which we are interested 'works'. It is not necessary to articulate a theory explicitly; in most aspects of our lives, we do not. But the potential penalty for the failure to be explicit is to carry forward mistaken assumptions or inconsistent arguments. As the economist John Maynard Keynes (1936) (whose own theories waned during the 1970s and 1980s but may now be undergoing a modest revival) said:

> Practical men, who believe themselves to be quite exempt from any intellectual influences, are usually the slaves of some defunct economist.

We prefer, therefore, to be explicit in our theorising even though the main text does not relate our views to the work of other authors.[1] That is the purpose of this chapter.

Why, therefore, is much of this chapter, indeed, much of the book, about the past? Theories of the future, unless wholly speculative, must rely on a knowledge of the past. They assume that past relationships between what are considered to be relevant variables will continue to hold, at least to some extent. This does not, of course, mean that the future will simply be similar to, or develop incrementally from, the past; relationships between variables may change, sometimes quickly, and indeed the late twentieth century has often been dubbed the 'age of discontinuity'. But these discontinuities are still likely to be the result of the interaction of known variables. A final word about the content of our theorizing here; on the face of it, we employ two rather different kinds of variables. The first kind is ostensibly objective and measurable, for example economic, demographic, and technological changes. The second kind of variable is 'soft': ideology, attitudes and opinions. But it is not necessary to push very hard for this distinction to disappear; objective variables such as technology only have significance for decision-making in so far as they are endowed with it by the opinions of sufficient relevant players.[2]

**THE SUPPLY SIDE**

By definition, the resources available in any country at any particular time are finite. In the case of the UK, therefore, the NHS is in competition with other potential areas of expenditure for the resources which it uses. The conventional measure of the resources immediately available to a country is its gross domestic product (GDP), roughly definable as the aggregate final value of goods and services produced domestically. Expenditure on health services, whether public or private, takes a share of this, currently about 6 per cent in the UK, but much more in some other countries, notably the USA. Most UK governments seek macroeconomic policies (policies for managing the whole economy) which will cause the real GDP to grow as rapidly as possible, since this is what enables the satisfaction of most economic, and therefore political demands. The question, of course, is how to do this; here we enter the world of macroeconomic theory. For some 60 years now, public expenditure has been seen as a crucial factor for real economic growth (i.e. growth of the GDP), though, as we shall see, in some very different ways. And because, in the case of the UK, public expenditure on health care (i.e. the NHS) accounts for more than 85 per cent of all health care spending, the NHS is very much implicated in macro-economic policy.

From immediately after the Second World War, public expenditure was believed to be an important macroeconomic lever for stimulating economic growth. During periods of low growth, an increase in public expenditure would help to stimulate demand by increasing levels of employment, though at times of rapid economic growth such a policy would not be appropriate since it would tend to increase inflation. We have already made a reference to the decline in credibility of this 'Keynesian' economic model; though Keynes always had his opponents, the beginning of this decline can probably be dated as the oil crisis of the early 1970s. Since that time, macroeconomic orthodoxy has increasingly been dominated by theories which see public expenditure in a more hostile light.

These alternative theories (various versions of what are usually termed 'monetarism' and 'supply-side' economics) point out that public expenditure can only be financed in one or more of three ways, all of which have deleterious effects on economic growth. One way is to expand the money supply by printing money and/or increasing the availability of credit; as is well known, monetarists believe that this always drives up inflation. A second approach is for government to borrow money (by, for instance, selling securities), the effect of which, it is held by 'supply-siders', is to drive up interest rates generally and thus discourage private investment and/or increase inflation. Further, monetarists believe that such government debt functions as quasi-money in the banking system (i.e. the banks lend on the strength of it) and is therefore inflationary. The final approach is to increase taxation; here, the 'supply-siders' argue, the result is to reduce incentives to work, to take entre-preneurial risks, or to save.[3]

The most important early manifestation of this change in economic orthodoxy was the introduction in the mid-1970s (by a Labour Government, note) of the 'cash limits' system of finance for the UK public sector.[4] Instead of the previous system, in which the volume of public services was protected by a policy of compensating public sector agencies for actual wage and price inflation, there was developed an alternative by which the agencies themselves were made to carry the risk of inflation over and above a figure predicted by the Government at the beginning of the financial year. Such a system has the consequence that inflation in excess of the prediction leads, all other things equal, to a reduction in the real resources available to the public agency in question. Since expectations of inflation are to some extent self-fulfilling, or even self-exceeding (for instance, they help to underpin trade union pay claims and manufacturers' price decisions), and since inflation will itself increase public expenditure, there is an obvious temptation for governments to *underestimate*, though sometimes this has to be made good in mid-financial year, as occurred, for instance as a result of the costs of the nurses' and midwives' clinical grading structure, introduced in 1988. It has been the policy of governments to extend the proportion of total public expenditure subject to such cash limits, which reached 64 per cent by 1990. Social security expenditure contains the largest single element of *non*-cash-limited resource; it is difficult to limit, because of people's statutory entitlement to unemployment and sickness benefits, retirement pensions, and so on.

At various points in the 1980s, these economic theories have led to two Government macroeconomic objectives which affect public expenditure. The first has been to reduce, and if possible eliminate, the public sector borrowing requirement (PSBR), that is, the excess of government spending over revenue. This was achieved from 1986 to 1990, prior to the General Election of April 1992 but the PSBR was estimated at £28 billion, that is, something approaching the total cost of the NHS, for 1992–93 and was forecast to remain in existence at least until 1994. The estimate was subsequently revised upwards to £37 billion, and at the time of writing the PSBR seems likely to exceed even this figure. The second macroeconomic objective has been to reduce the proportion of GDP occupied by public expenditure; in the event, this fell from over 47 per cent in 1982 to some 39.5 per cent in 1990. It is easy to see how both of these objectives necessitate the control of public expenditure. In the second case, it must be controlled by definition. In the first, it is its relationship with government revenue that has to be controlled.

The reader will have noted that we have now occupied several paragraphs with a discussion of public expenditure in general, without any mention of the NHS. Why does control of the former necessitate control of the latter? In principle, it does not; it would be possible to re-order government priorities, so as to take resources

**Table 2.1** Shares of government expenditure by selected function (percentages of Planning Total: outturn)

| Expenditure on | 1978–79 | 1980–81 | 1982–83 | 1984–85 | 1986–87 | 1988–89 | 1990–91 | 1992–93 (planned) |
|---|---|---|---|---|---|---|---|---|
| Social Security | 25 | 25 | 29 | 30 | 34 | 34 | 31 | 31 |
| Education & Science | 12 | 12 | 11 | 13 | 15 | 16 | 15 | 17 |
| Defence | 11 | 12 | 13 | 13 | 13 | 13 | 12 | 11 |
| Health & Personal Social Services (England) | 11 | 12 | 12 | 13 | 14 | 16 | 15 | 15 |

*Sources:* 1978–83, Cm 9143 The Government's Expenditure Plans 1984–85 to 1986–87 (1984); 1984–93, Cm 1913 The Government's Expenditure Plans 1992–93 to 1994–95 (1992).

from (say) defence or social security and give them to health. Table 2.1 sets out the distribution of UK public expenditure between major programmes.

By 1986, social security represented some one-third of all public expenditure. Moreover, as noted above, the bulk of this huge proportion is not cash-limited and is not, therefore, subject to ready control. The next largest areas of public expenditure after social security, where the burden of control necessarily falls, are health, defence and education. In terms of Table 2.1, therefore, the NHS can be regarded as fortunate in having grown; indeed Table 2.1 can be interpreted as a movement of resources from defence into health. We shall see, however, in the final section of this chapter that this does not necessarily mean that the NHS has always been fully funded in accordance with its 'needs'.

## THE DEMAND SIDE

In this section we discuss four main areas of demand pressure upon the NHS: demographic changes, technological development, the costs of increasing efficiency in hospital usage and public opinion. A preliminary point should be noted. Our mixture is of 'objective' and 'subjective' variables: the crucial common factor is policymakers' awareness of, and concern, about them. Without such awareness and concern, they would not count towards our explanation of why governments have come to perceive a need to control health professionals.

We begin, then, by looking at demographic change, summarized in Table 2.2. The key point here is the increase in the numbers of elderly persons in the UK population, both in absolute terms and as a percentage of the total. Reflecting a long-term decline in the birth rate and increase in life expectancy, the proportion of the population aged 75 years and over grew from 4.2 per cent in 1961 to 6.9 per cent in 1990. It will plateau at 7.4 per cent around the year 2001, though the 85 years and over age group will continue to increase.[5] The significance of these population groups is their expense in terms of NHS utilization: Figure 2.1 indicates this clearly.

Very roughly, the costs to the NHS of providing services to this increasingly elderly population amounts to between 0.5 and 1 per cent per annum (in real terms) of the total budget of health authorities, a figure conceded by the Government. The detailed figures are set out in Figure 2.2.

**Table 2.2** Recent demographic trends (thousands) in the United Kingdom, according to age groups

| Mid-year | All ages | Under 1 | 1–4 | 5–14 | 15–24 | 25–34 | 35–44 | 45–59 | 60–64 | 65–74 | 75–84 | 85 and over |
|---|---|---|---|---|---|---|---|---|---|---|---|---|
| 1961 | 52 807 | 912 | 3362 | 8085 | 7056 | 6655 | 7137 | 10 605 | 2788 | 3977 | 1885 | 346 |
| 1971 | 55 928 | 899 | 3654 | 8916 | 8144 | 6971 | 6512 | 10 202 | 3222 | 4764 | 2160 | 485 |
| 1981 | 56 352 | 730 | 2725 | 8147 | 9019 | 8010 | 6774 | 9540 | 2935 | 5194 | 2676 | 602 |
| 1986 | 56 763 | 749 | 2893 | 7157 | 9263 | 8024 | 7719 | 9220 | 3055 | 5005 | 2969 | 709 |
| 1987 | 56 930 | 758 | 2928 | 7062 | 9162 | 8210 | 7810 | 9204 | 2983 | 5038 | 3016 | 760 |
| 1988 | 57 065 | 779 | 2968 | 7013 | 8977 | 8387 | 7853 | 9264 | 2940 | 5031 | 3056 | 796 |
| 1989 | 57 236 | 771 | 3037 | 7017 | 8730 | 8590 | 7870 | 9358 | 2910 | 5021 | 3098 | 835 |
| 1990 | 57 411 | 775 | 3066 | 7079 | 8473 | 8805 | 7890 | 9438 | 2896 | 5008 | 3114 | 866 |

*Source:* OPCS, *Population Trends*, No. 67, 1992, p. 41.

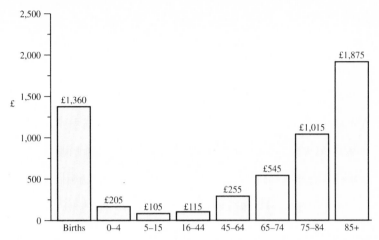

**Figure 2.1** Hospitals and community health services gross current expenditure per head 1989–90 (estimate)

*Source:* Cm 1913 (1992).

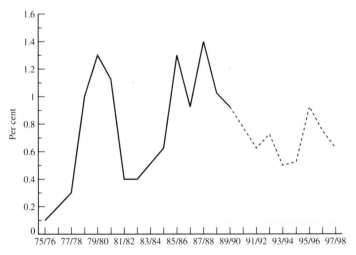

**Figure 2.2** Estimated growth in demand for HCHS from demographic changes. Increase over previous year

*Source:* Cm 1913 (1992).

Next, health care technology: by this, we mean not only high-technology 'hardware' and drugs, but health care techniques, including packages of care, more generally. Despite our broad definition, it happens to be the case that efforts to calculate the costs of development have concentrated on the former area. Much depends on how the calculation is performed; we quote two extreme comparisons to illustrate this. In 1984 a pair of American academics published their calculation of the cost of raising UK utilization rates of 11 specific technologies (bone-marrow transplantation, chemotherapy for cancer, computed tomography scanning, coronary artery bypass grafts, diagnostic radiology, renal dialysis, haemophilia treatments, total hip replacement, radiotherapy, total parenteral nutrition and intensive care) to then current US utilization rates. The result would have been an increase in NHS expenditure of more than 12 per cent. At the other extreme lies the British Government estimate (Robinson and Judge 1987):

> [for the financial year 1986–87] increases in activity arising from medical advance are estimated to absorb in the region of half a percent of resources annually.

Two further points need to be borne in mind when considering expenditure on health care technology.[6] First, none of the above figures contains any allowance for the development of 'soft' technology such as new models of (community) care for the mentally ill or persons with learning difficulties. As Klein (1989) has noted:

> Even if the limitations of medical technology in curing disease and disability are now becoming apparent, there are no such limitations on the scope of health services for providing care for those who cannot be cured. Even if policies of prevention and social engineering were to be successfully introduced, their very success in extending life expectancy would create new demands for alleviating the chronic degenerative diseases of old age. In other words, no policy can ensure that people will drop dead painlessly at the age of 80, not having troubled the health services previously.

Second, the utilization of technologies is more in the hands of health care professionals, especially doctors, than is commonly imagined;

here is one researcher's description of the development of screening for spina bifida (Stocking 1985):

> . . . innovations . . . may have diffused readily because there was no need to define explicitly the uses to which staff and equipment were being put. For example, neural tube defect screening with its various components of blood tests, amniocentesis, counselling and abortion is costly. However, it seems to have been able to diffuse relatively rapidly because in its initial stages in any particular locality, no new equipment or funds needed to be requested. It is only as the service builds up that it becomes necessary to ask for additional laboratory equipment, etc.

Our third source of demand for health care resources can be labelled the 'efficiency trap'. This label refers to the fact that, outside psychiatry, the NHS has been 'treating more patients' than ever before, and that even though it has been treating them more efficiently, there is still an additional cost to be borne. Consider the following:

- Between 1978 and 1986, the number of non-psychiatric beds available fell by some 16 per cent. In the same period, the number of patients treated in them increased by some 19 per cent.
- Self-evidently, this entails either or both of shorter lengths of stay and less unoccupied bed time. In the event, lengths of stay over the above period fell by around 24 per cent.
- Since the length of a hospital stay is a major determinant of its cost, one would expect a fall here (i.e. an increase in efficiency, albeit in a rather narrow sense) and as Figure 2.3 shows one did indeed occur.
- But acute inpatients do not incur constant daily costs; much variable expenditure (such as pathology tests, X-rays, and surgical operations) is highest in the early part of the stay. As a consequence, costs per case fell, not by 24 per cent, but by something in excess of 15 per cent

The result of all this is that, despite improvements in efficiency, the costs of the additional inpatient cases outweighed the saving by about 1.2 per cent. Official figures, however, claim overall cash-releasing efficiency *savings* in the region of 0.7 per cent per annum. It follows from the above that savings must have been made in the psychiatric and non-inpatient sectors of the Service.[7]

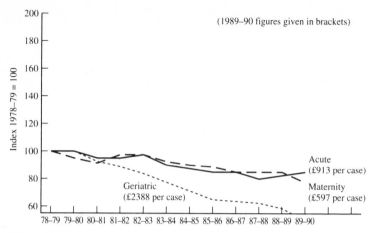

**Figure 2.3**   Hospital unit costs
*Source:* Cm 1913 (1992).


The fourth and final source of demand to which we wish to refer is from the public. Crudely expressed, there is substantial opinion poll evidence which suggests three things. First, a large proportion of the public believe that too little money is spent on the NHS; a smaller proportion, though still an absolute majority, believe that additional revenue should come from central taxation. Second, the NHS is the most popular sector of the welfare state, both in the sense that public support for the service in general is very high (over 90 per cent), and that satisfaction levels amongst users are high (in the 80 per cent range). Third, polls of public opinion concerning the respective esteem of different occupations consistently place doctors and nurses in the top two or three places.

We know that, whatever reservations one might have about the meaning of poll data, politicians are aware of, and concerned about, the findings. At the very least, one would expect governments to be cautious about how they are seen to deal with issues of NHS finance and of managing professionals. It is not accidental that Mrs Thatcher declared the NHS to be 'safe in our hands', or that NHS ancillary (rather than professional) staff were the first to feel the brunt of managerial strategies such as competitive tendering.[8]

It is, however, the addition to these factors of one further feature of UK health care that turns them into such an intractable problem

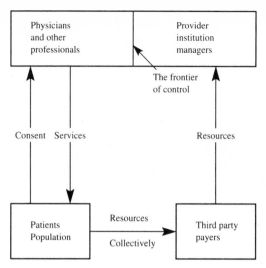

**Figure 2.4**    Third party payment for health care

*Source:* Adapted from S. Harrison (1988) *Managing the NHS*. Chapman and Hall, London.

for government. Since (like in many other countries) health care is largely free at the point of delivery, it is to be expected that people will always want more of it than is supplied. Health care will therefore have to be rationed; and it will be upon those who fund it (in the UK context, government), upon whom that burden falls. This is illustrated in Figure 2.4.

The generic name for the type of health system illustrated in Figure 2.4 is *third party payment*. The defining feature of such a system is that payment for services is divorced from receipt of them. This is achieved by a third party collecting resources from the population (effectively pooling the risks of needing health care) and redirecting the resources to the providers of care in hospitals and other institutions, or, more precisely, to the managers of such institutions. As we have noted, the third party in the UK context is central government, collecting resources via the tax system; in other countries, the third parties might be insurance organizations, or sick funds, collecting resources via premiums or contributions deducted from pay.

Much of our discussion of demand for health care can be summarized in two *general* statements about the type of system illustrated in

Figure 2.4. First, patients have little or no disincentive to maximize the amount of care that they demand, because it is (largely) free, though it may carry non-monetary costs such as time, inconvenience, or discomfort. 'Certainly', a thoughtful patient would conclude, 'my care has to be paid for, but spread out across a population, my share will be negligible'. The jargon term for this is *moral hazard*. Of course, if many or all of the population behave in this way, the costs will not be negligible. Second, providers of health care have few incentives to do other than maximize the amount of care which they provide; the patient does not have to pay, and there will be no bad debts. Hence the normal supply/demand 'scissors' of the economic textbook are no longer present. This is called *supplier-induced demand* and may arise from situations where health care professionals are paid by item of service, or from a desire to try out new technology, or simply from a desire to help the patient. Of course, there are constraints, such as the provider's own time.

Both these general statements can be exaggerated as predictors of the behaviour of individual patients or professionals, but it is easy to see the pressures that the tendencies that they describe place on a health service. Specifically, they place much of the burden of controlling the system upon the third party payer, since no-one else has much incentive to do so. In the UK, this is government, whose interests in controlling public expenditure we have already discussed.

The process of controlling expenditure amounts to rationing health care, the topic of our next section.

## RATIONING UK HEALTH CARE

It should be clear from what we have already said in this chapter that rationing of medical care is a chronic necessity. If there is finite supply and no obvious limitation to demand, then some people who desire health care will not get it. What this necessity does not, however, determine is the form which rationing takes. More precisely, *who* makes the decisions, what *criteria* are used, and what *processes* are employed?[9]

Even though, as we have shown, NHS rationing pressures have been particularly intense in the last few years, the necessity is not new. The NHS has rationed health care since its inception but by means that were very much diffused and largely implicit. Because of the system of global funding by government, it was possible for *overall* financial control to be maintained without giving detailed direction on how money was to be spent. Government did play a part, as did managers, especially with regard to expenditure on major capital items and new consultant posts, and charges for prescriptions and dentistry, but the main burden of rationing was left to be performed by doctors themselves; it is only a modest exaggeration to say that doctors were allowed to do whatever they wished so long as the allocated sum was not exceeded. *Some* of these medical decisions were explicit, in the form of hospital waiting lists, but the majority were implicit, in the form of clinical decisions: in other words, the exercise of 'clinical freedom'. The point is well made, albeit in the dramatic context of a potentially fatal condition, by the following quotation from two American researchers of the NHS (Aaron and Schwartz 1984: 101):

> By various means, physicians . . . try to make the denial of care seem routine or optimal. Confronted by a person older than the prevailing unofficial age of cut-off for dialysis, the British GP tells the victim of chronic renal failure or his family that nothing can be done except to make the patient as comfortable as possible in the time remaining. The British nephrologist tells the family of a patient who is difficult to handle that dialysis would be painful and burdensome and that the patient would be more comfortable without it.

As we suggested in our discussion of the third notion of professionalism (Chapter 1), such an arrangement is highly convenient for the state. Why, therefore, should a government wish to change things? The answer is that such arrangements require the acquiescence of doctors; in the past, such acquiescence was generally forthcoming, for at least two reasons. First, for many clinicians, the process was largely an unconscious one; their assessments of patients' thresholds of 'need' shifted with the availability of resources. Second, for those for whom the process was a conscious one, optimism that resource availability would continue to grow was sufficient to prevent too much discontent.

But, in the early 1980s, both of these two factors began to be affected by the Government's perception that there was a particularly acute crisis of public expenditure. Growth in health care expenditure was to be cut back, and many commentators inter-preted this as an absolute cut. At the same time, there was a good deal of talk about possible alternative financing methods for the NHS. As a result, few doctors could continue in unconscious rationing, or with any immediate optimism that substantial real growth was imminent. Proposals to review the financing base of the NHS were abandoned by the Government in mid-1983. And its early aspirations that private expenditure on health care would soon grow to 25 per cent of the UK total were disappointed.[10] A new approach to rationing had, therefore, to emerge. Other than the politically dangerous reliance on changes for services, at least three logical possibilities existed for such a new approach, and all were attempted in varying degrees.

One approach was to ration explicitly by making a Government decision that certain services would not be available 'on the NHS'. Although certain services (i.e. parts of what is now termed 'complementary medicine') had always been defined out of the NHS simply by virtue of their *practitioners* not being recognized, this explicit approach has two grave disadvantages from a govern-ment perspective. For a start it breached the statutory basis of the NHS (National Health Service Act, 1946, S.1(1), emphasis added):

> It shall be the duty of the Minister . . . to promote the establishment . . . of a *comprehensive* health service designed to secure improvement in the physical and mental health of the people . . . and the prevention, diagnosis and treatment of illness . . .

Moreover, it was likely to be politically unpopular; it is one thing for a Secretary of State to be aware that (to return to an example that we used before) access to renal dialysis is in practice governed by an age cut-off, but quite something else to announce it as government policy. In the event, therefore, this first alternative approach to rationing was attempted, though successfully, only in the form of restrictions on prescribing certain proprietary drugs, which were implemented in 1984.

The second possible new approach to rationing was to tighten implicit rationing by purporting to cut out waste. Such a policy has the great advantage that it is difficult to criticize in principle; we are all, in principle, in favour of cutting out waste just as (as the late George Woodcock is reputed to have observed) we are all against sin. And this approach was attempted, too, in the NHS and elsewhere in the public services. From 1981 onwards, the NHS was expected to make 'efficiency savings'; this practice consisted of assuming that health authorities' outturn expenditure would be less than their nominal budget by a specified (between 0.2 and 0.5) percentage, and hence providing an actual budget to match only the assumed outturn. Since the arrangement provided no controls over where savings were made, it was no more than a convenient assumption that they resulted from improved efficiency rather than cuts in services. It may, therefore, be ingenuous, or disingenuous to assume that service cuts will not occur, and indeed subsequent evidence from the National Audit Office suggests that they did.[11] The efficiency savings notion was transformed into the post-Griffiths Report 'cost-improvement programmes' and became incorporated into our third possible alternative approach to rationing.

This third approach was to strengthen the management of the NHS: to turn managers into agents of central government as a means of controlling professional behaviour. In terms of Figure 2.4, this would represent a shift in the 'frontier of control' between managers and professionals: an erosion of professional autonomy. Such an approach would have at least two major advantages. It would be able to trade upon an increasing public willingness to engage in critical questioning about professional activity, despite the continued esteem in which doctors and nurses were held, and to which we have already referred. More important, it would allow government to adopt an ambiguous posture towards NHS efficiency. On the one hand it would be able to argue that, in strengthening management it was ensuring the credibility of its efficiency strategy by providing people who could control the origin of savings. On the other hand, it could evade blame for actual problems that became evident at operational level by arguing that the facility for better management had been provided and that it was up to managers to get on with it. This general tendency of governments has been neatly summed up by Klein (1983: 140):

> . . . while in the post-war era of economic growth governments were anxious to centralise credit – to claim responsibility for the improvements made possible by increasing prosperity – the stress now is on diffusing blame for the inevitable shortcomings in an era of economic crisis: to decentralise responsibility is also to disclaim blame.

As most readers will be well aware, it is this third strategy which has formed the Government's main approach to the problems of the NHS during the 1980s and early 1990s. Its defining features are a reduction in the autonomy of doctors, and the creation of a unified management hierarchy at the expense of the individual hierarchies of the other health professions. It began with the creation of the regional review process and performance indicators in 1982, continued through the establishment of general management (together with its associated incentives and sanctions and the development of resource management) and has recently been strengthened by being placed within the context of a purchaser/provider split and a process of contracting for health care. This third strategy is the subject of this book: controlling health professionals.

It is necessary to add a caveat about the nature of the explanation which we have constructed, of how the necessity to control health professionals came about. We have concentrated upon the macro-level pressures which have brought about this necessity; we have also argued that these pressures are relatively long-run in character, for which reason we shall be returning to their future effect in Chapter 6. But explaining this *general* necessity to control professionals is not the same as explaining how the *detailed* policy choices about (say) performance indicators, or general management, occurred. Such detailed explanations are very much concerned with the micro-level of activity: personalities and short-term political pressures. We give a flavour of these in each of the Chapters, 3, 4 and 5, which follow.

## PUBLIC EXPENDITURE AND THE NHS: FUTURE PROSPECTS

In order to make an assessment of future prospects for public expenditure and its impact on the NHS, we need to look in a little detail both at public expenditure trends in general, and in the NHS in particular.

First, the general picture, as touched upon in the first section of this chapter, is set out in greater detail in Table 2.3.

Column (1) shows what can be regarded as total public expenditure (including health and social services) as a percentage of GDP. (It should be noted that about half of this is taken up in 'transfer

**Table 2.3** Public sector finance: 1979–93

| Financial Year (GDP by calendar year) | (1) General government expenditure as percentage of Gross Domestic Product | (2) Public Sector Borrowing Requirement (excl. privatization proceeds) | (3) PSBR (excl. privatization proceeds) as percentage of GDP | (4) Privatization proceeds (£ billion) | (5) PSBR (£ billion) | (6) PSBR as percentage of GDP | (7) Current surplus as percentage of GDP |
|---|---|---|---|---|---|---|---|
| 1978–79 | 43.2 | 9.2 | 5.3 | – | 9.2 | 5.3 | 1.8 |
| 1979–80 | 43.4 | 10.3 | 4.9 | 0.4 | 9.9 | 4.8 | 2.1 |
| 1980–81 | 45.4 | 12.7 | 5.3 | 0.2 | 12.5 | 5.3 | 0.4 |
| 1981–82 | 46.4 | 9.1 | 3.5 | 0.5 | 8.6 | 3.3 | 2.3 |
| 1982–83 | 46.6 | 9.4 | 3.3 | 0.5 | 8.9 | 3.1 | 2.0 |
| 1983–84 | 45.6 | 10.8 | 3.5 | 1.1 | 9.7 | 3.1 | 1.6 |
| 1984–85 | 46.0 | 12.1 | 3.6 | 2.0 | 10.1 | 3.0 | 0.7 |
| 1985–86 | 44.3 | 8.3 | 2.3 | 2.7 | 5.6 | 1.5 | 1.8 |
| 1986–87 | 43.1 | 8.1 | 2.1 | 4.5 | 3.6 | 0.9 | 1.0 |
| 1987–88 | 41.0 | 1.7 | 0.4 | 5.1 | –3.4 | – | 2.2 |
| 1988–89 | 38.6 | –7.5 | – | 7.1 | –14.6 | – | 3.9 |
| 1989–90 | 39.0 | –3.7 | – | 4.2 | –7.9 | – | 3.9 |
| 1990–91 | 40.1 | 4.8 | 0.9 | 5.3 | –0.5 | – | 2.8 |
| 1991–92 | 41.9 | 21.7 | 3.7 | 7.9 | 13.7 | 2.4 | 0.1 |
| 1992–93 (est.) | 44.7 | 45.0 | 7.5 | 8.0 | 37.0 | 6.2 | –1.8 |

*Sources:*

Col. (1): calculated from *Autumn Statement*, 1992, Cm 2096.
Col. (2): calculated from Cm 2096.
Col. (3): CSO, *Annual Abstract of Statistics*, 1991 and 1992.
Col. (4): Cm 2096.
Col. (7): *The Guardian*, 23 March 1992.

payments' such as social security payments, as opposed to government spending on goods and services.) Columns (2) and (3) in effect show the difference between this sum and government income: the PSBR, as a cash sum, and as a percentage of GDP. (The negative figures indicate a surplus, or public sector debt repayment.) The deficit, which has escalated rapidly in the last two years, has been somewhat ameliorated by the receipts shown in Column (4), that is the Government's proceeds from the sale of state-owned industries such as British Telecom and the water boards. These receipts partially offset the deficit, leaving the net PSBR shown in cash terms in Column (5) and as a percentage of GDP in Column (6). The PSBR's existence has typically been due to *capital* (as opposed to current, or revenue, expenditure), so that if the former is omitted, a surplus emerges. These figures are shown in Column (7). We wish to draw out four important points.

First, the Government's policy objectives in relation to public expenditure have proved elusive; neither the reduction of expenditure as a proportion of GDP, nor the reduction/elimination of the deficit has been sustained. Second, the deficit (PSBR) is now very large; even after offsetting privatization receipts; the 1992–93 estimate of £37 billion comfortably exceeds the total cost of the NHS. Third, the negative figures at the foot of Column (7) implies that the Government is now borrowing to pay for current, as well as capital, expenditure. Finally, privatization proceeds are obviously finite (hence the cliche about 'selling the family silver') and at the time of writing are forecast to decline after the £8 billion peak in 1992–93.

The inevitable conclusion, it seems to us, will be an extremely difficult few years for public expenditure, a conclusion which is strengthened by the presence of a re-elected Government with a four or five year mandate. In order to assess the potential impact upon the NHS, we have constructed Figure 2.5. The solid line shows the annual real changes in the resource inputs to the NHS: cash increases plus cash-releasing efficiency savings (see above), all deflated by the NHS Pay and Prices Index.[12] It represents, in effect, the supply side of the balance sheet. The broken line shows the demand side: annual required changes resulting from demographic shift, and technological development (see above), though policy change has been excluded. The overall picture until 1990 is very much one of balance of supply and demand. But in the last two years there has been a considerable increase in supply compared with demand.

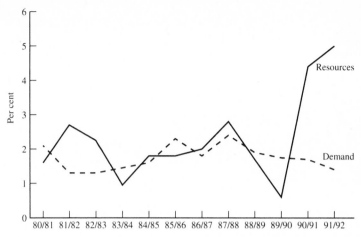

**Figure 2.5**   Health services growth. Resources are Cash + Efficiency deflated by NHS PPI; Demand is Demography + Technology

*Source:* Thunhurst and Harrison, *The Guardian*, 25 March 1992.

In the context of the probability of a restricted public expenditure over the next few years, it is our reading of the above data that the NHS is unlikely to receive large real funding increases. In such circumstances, the emphasis will be on the pursuit of efficiency, and hence on the control of health professionals.

# 3

# CHALLENGING THE PROFESSIONALS

## INTRODUCTION

In Chapter 1, we drew attention to the potential conflict between the notions of management and professionalism: the former as getting other people to do things, the latter as employing one's own judgement about what to do and how to do it. One obvious approach to this tension would be to attempt to resolve it by subordinating professional autonomy to managerial will: to challenge the professions 'head on' as it were. It is this direct form of challenge which provides the subject matter for this chapter. First, however, we need to establish some kind of 'starting line' for the relationships between managers and professionals. This we do by looking at the character of these relations up to the early 1980s.

## MANAGING THE NHS, 1966–82

One important source of information about how the NHS used to work is the findings of research projects. Research into the organization and management of the NHS hardly began until the mid-1960s (hence the title of this section) and did not produce a great volume of findings until the mid-1970s. As was indicated in Chapter 2, 1982 represented something of a watershed in thinking about NHS management, so that what follows here is a summary of research findings up to that date.

Although the approaches adopted towards this research were

quite varied, as were the scale and locations of the projects and the research methods employed, their findings were remarkably consistent. Whilst it is true that many studies found exceptions to the general summary which follows, these exceptions were in a small minority. We can summarize the research findings in four broad statements.

First, the shape of the total service provided by the NHS was the aggregate outcome of individual doctors' clinical decisions, rather than the result of decisions made by politicians, policymakers, planners or managers. These other actors had, of course, some influence over decisions about major new developments, such as hospitals or large items of technology, and, in the case of politicians and central policymakers, almost total influence about the extent and geographical distribution of finance. But it was clinical doctors who decided which patients to accept, how to investigate and treat them, whether to admit them to hospital, and how long to keep them there. Thus, contrary to the usual assumptions of 'textbook' management, managers were not the most influential actors in the organization; doctors were. It is important, however, not to misunderstand this statement. It was not due either to some conspiracy by doctors, nor due to the influence of a few, prominent individuals modelled upon Sir Lancelot Spratt. It was simply the result of doctors getting on with what they (and, as we shall see, everyone else) perceived to be their jobs.[1]

Our second statement describes the nature of managerial work in the pre-1982 NHS, and again contradicts the textbook model of the manager. Whilst the latter pictures (indeed, often *defines*) management as *pro-active*, as the pursuit of objectives, research shows the NHS manager to have been *reactive*. That is, managers' work, even at the most senior levels, was very much driven by problems, and, moreover, problems thrust upon the managers by other actors.

This leads directly to our third statement, since if managers' work was driven by problems we should ask about the nature and source of these problems. The research showed that the managers' problems came typically from *within* the organization rather than from outside it: from doctors, other professionals and from trade unions, rather than from patients, their relatives, the community at large or (after their creation in 1974) Community Health Councils. And many of the problems consisted in dealing with conflicts between or within the producer groups.

Finally, our fourth statement: the character of change in the pre-1982 NHS was *incremental*. By this, we refer to two related observations. The prevailing assumption about the pattern of services, and indeed about the services themselves, was that they were good or at least about right. As a result of this tendency to take the *status quo* for granted, there was almost no evaluation either of the pattern of resource distribution or of the quality, effectiveness, or efficiency of the services themselves. Instead, there was a strong tendency for the service to develop along the lines of 'more of the same', though with the inclusion of such new technologies as came along. This lack of root and branch evaluation is, once again, in sharp contrast to textbook models of management. However, a great deal of managerial effort *was* devoted to decisions about how to allocate the additional resources which (in the 1960s and 1970s) were available in most financial years. Much of this effort, as one might guess from our analysis so far, went into trying to reconcile or arbitrate competing professional demands for the resources.

To sum up the picture printed by the research findings, the pre-1982 NHS manager can be labelled a *diplomat*. Rather than being, as one might expect from the management textbooks, someone who shaped the NHS and controlled its direction, he or she helped to provide and organize the facilities and resources for professionals to get on with their work, and helped to mediate conflicts within the organization. The role is well summed up in both maintenance metaphors ('oiling the wheels', 'greasing the rails') and circus metaphors ('juggling the balls', 'keeping the plates spinning', 'riding two horses at once'). And, of course, the manager wasn't even *called* a manager officially. 'Administrator' was probably the most common formal title, though they would often have described themselves as managers.[2]

In hindsight, it is easy to pour ridicule on the manager-as-diplomat: to characterize it as weak and ineffective management. Following the Griffiths Report's 1983 diagnosis of what then seemed to be wrong with NHS management (which bears a remarkable similarity to our four statements above), such a view has been commonplace in and around the Service. But two points should be borne in mind.

First, hindsight is hindsight. It is only since about 1982, just before the Griffiths Report, that the 'diplomat' model has been seen to be inappropriate. Prior to that time, it was not merely how NHS managers actually behaved, but also represented how they were *supposed* to behave. In its time, it represented a prescription, springing from the view that professional autonomy was the appro-priate foundation for a national health service (see the above quotation from *Patients First*.) And, crucially, this view was en-shrined in the formal organization structures of the period. This can be seen at its clearest in the 1974 system of consensus decision-making by multidisciplinary management teams.[3]

The consensus team model contained, and to a large extent formalized, all four elements of the 'diplomat' model, though, as we have made clear, these elements were not novel. Medical influence was institutionalized through the presence of three doctors, one appointed and two elected by their clinical colleagues, on the management team at the operational (District) level. The formal remit of the team was defined as matters that were beyond the responsibility of any single member; although this did not of itself preclude pro-active behaviour, the outcome was that teams were frequently a forum for information passing and for deciding how issues and problems should be handled. A consensus rule for decision-making implied that each team member had a veto; the predictable effect of this was to reinforce incremental decision-making. Any team member whose services were threatened could veto change. Finally, the fact that the team's membership was *defined* in professional terms, and that it had no remit to represent the consumer (this function having been transferred to Community Health Councils), meant that it adopted a viewpoint very much based on that of NHS employees. It was *producer-oriented* rather than consumer-oriented.

One way of summing all this up would be to say that medical autonomy was the single factor that led to many of the phenomena that we have observed. In such a situation it would hardly be expected that managers would be the most influential actors. More-over, if doctors were clinically autonomous, claims to autonomy made by other professions could not easily be realised without some dilution of medical autonomy. For the non-medical professions, therefore, the pursuit of their own management arrangements was often seen as a better strategy for occupational self-control than a direct claim to their own clinical autonomy, which might bring them into confrontation with the doctors. In such a situation, reactive management and a producer orientation was almost inevitable. And in these circumstances there was little incentive to pursue evaluation or critical review of the producers' activities.

Secondly, it is necessary to remember that such 'diplomatic'

**Table 3.1**   International comparisons of health care expenditure (percentage of GDP at market prices, 1990)

| Country | Public expenditure on health | Total expenditure on health |
|---|---|---|
| Australia | 5.2 | 7.5 |
| Austria | 5.6 | 8.4 |
| Belgium | 6.1 | 7.4 |
| Canada | 6.7 | 9.0 |
| Denmark | 5.2 | 6.2 |
| Finland | 6.2 | 7.4 |
| France | 6.6 | 8.9 |
| Germany | 5.9 | 8.1 |
| Greece | 4.0 | 5.3 |
| Ireland | 5.8 | 7.1 |
| Italy | 5.9 | 7.6 |
| Japan | 4.9 | 6.5 |
| Netherlands | 5.9 | 8.1 |
| New Zealand | 5.9 | 7.2 |
| Norway | 6.9 | 7.2 |
| Portugal | 4.1 | 6.7 |
| Spain | 5.2 | 6.6 |
| Sweden | 7.8 | 8.7 |
| Switzerland | 5.1 | 7.4 |
| United Kingdom | 5.2 | 6.1 |
| United States | 5.2 | 12.4 |

*Source:* Office of Health Economics, *Compendium of Health Statistics 1992*, Tables 2.3 and 2.6.

management should not be equated with the complete absence of control over professionals. From its inception, long before the days of cash limits, the NHS's total budget and that of the agencies within it (e.g. health authorities) has been tightly controlled by central government, even though the nature of expenditure within the budget has not. This is one reason that it has been possible to maintain UK health expenditure at a relatively low level (expressed as a percentage of GDP) compared with other developed countries. This is illustrated in Table 3.1.

## BEYOND THE MANAGER AS DIPLOMAT

We now move to the post-1982 period, during which the diplomat model was rather rapidly discarded. In its place, the Government attempted to substitute a more pro-active vision of management, to create a new managerial cadre which would challenge the claims to autonomy made by professional groups within the NHS. In the first two chapters we have already reviewed the main influences which encouraged ministers to go down this road. These were the need to curb further increases in public expenditure (Chapter 2) and the belief that public services management had hitherto been wasteful, ineffective and unresponsive to service users (Chapter 1).

However, the reform of NHS management was more easily said than done. In the remainder of this chapter we examine *one* approach – that of directly challenging professional groups. Within this, three more specific strategies are discussed:

- Introducing general management
- Improving management information
- Weakening trade unions and professional associations

In the two subsequent chapters we deal with two quite different approaches – incorporating professionals into management roles (Chapter 4) and fundamentally restructuring the environment within which professionals operate (Chapter 5).

## GENERAL MANAGEMENT

According to Drucker (1955: 208):

> Most organisation theorists seem to believe that the one-man [*sic*] chief executive is a law of nature, requiring no proof and admitting of no doubt.

Though Drucker, one of the most influential management writers, argued that in practice many of the most successfully managed corporations had an executive *team* rather than a single chief executive, it seems that beliefs attributed to 'organization theorists' are as prevalent amongst managers today as they were in the 1950s. Indeed, the fact that the single chief executive, with the title of 'general manager' (GM) has only arrived in the NHS during the last decade is often treated as *prima facie* evidence of the Service's previous backwardness.

This is typified in (the then Mr) Roy Griffiths' much quoted observation (NHS Management Inquiry 1983: 12):

> In short, if Florence Nightingale were carrying her lamp through the corridors of the NHS today she would almost certainly be searching for the people in charge.

As we shall see, Mr Griffiths and his colleagues went on to recommend (and gain acceptance for) the introduction of general managers to the NHS. We shall also see that they were not the first people to have this idea. But first we need to examine the argument that lies behind the assertion that general managers are vital.

In practice, the assertion contains at least three quite separate assumptions. One is that any organization which is to survive has to engage in a reasonably coordinated set of activities. This is difficult to dispute, except to say that coordination (or general management) does not necessarily require general managers: there are alternative models, at least one of which (consensus teams) was widespread in the NHS at the time of the Griffiths inquiry.

A second assumption concerns individual accountability: the notion that one person should be answerable for effecting defined organizational tasks.[4] The implied argument here runs that only if an individual feels personally at risk in some way will he or she be motivated to see that the 'right' things actually get done. Apart from representing a rather crude view of human motivation, this carries the further implication that there exists some authoritative view of what constitutes 'the right thing'. Although this *could* mean accountability to the members of the organization, or to the users of the organization's products or services, in practice it usually means hierarchical accountability. Thus, arguments about *accountability* in organizations run straight into arguments about *control*.

This is the third argument which underpins the assertion that a chief executive is crucial: the fear that without such a role, people in the organization will 'do their own thing'. In the specific context of health service organizations, this is expressed especially as a concern to control professionals; that is, it adopts the second ('occupational control') of the three views of professionalism that we set out in Chapter 1.

Probably the earliest call for a general manager or chief executive was the Porritt Report, produced on behalf of the BMA in 1962. This report used the term 'administrator' and asserted that this individual should be medically qualified. Shortly afterwards, in

1966 the official Scottish Farquharson-Lang Report recommended that health authorities should employ a 'chief executive' who need not necessarily be medically qualified. This recommendation was not acted upon, and indeed was suppressed when the Report was publicized in England. Nevertheless, there was support from south of the border: in 1967, a joint working party of the (then) Institute of Hospital Administrators and the King's Fund argued (King Edward's Hospital Fund for London 1967: 24):

> that someone had to be in command of the [hospital] with authority over all the rest of the staff.

In the meantime, the NHS was moving in the opposite direction. In 1974 the NHS, along with local government, underwent a major reorganization. Rather than employing a chief executive or general manager, management at most levels of the service was to be conducted by multidisciplinary management teams; their composition, and their place in the organization, is shown in Figure 3.1.

Management at Regional, Area and District levels was conducted by multidisciplinary management teams in which individual team members were to have personal responsibility for their own spheres of work, but decisions which were multidisciplinary or strategic were handled collectively. The mode of decision-making by such teams was to be consensus; decisions needed the agreement of each of the team members. There was no authority relationship between teams at different levels, only between the Authorities themselves, with team members responsible to their respective Authorities. Moreover, several of the health professions which were not represented on the consensus team were nevertheless directly responsible to the Authority, and entitled to attend team meetings for the discussion of relevant issues. The relationship *between* teams was intended to be one of 'monitoring': the higher level possessing the right to give advice and obtain information but not directly to instruct the lower level. Disagreements either between teams, or amongst members of a particular team, were to be settled by reference to the appropriate Health Authority, though there was in practice a reluctance to adopt this procedure. (In Scotland and Wales there were some differences of terminology, and District teams in these countries were managerially accountable to area teams; Scottish teams did not include elected clinicians.)[5]

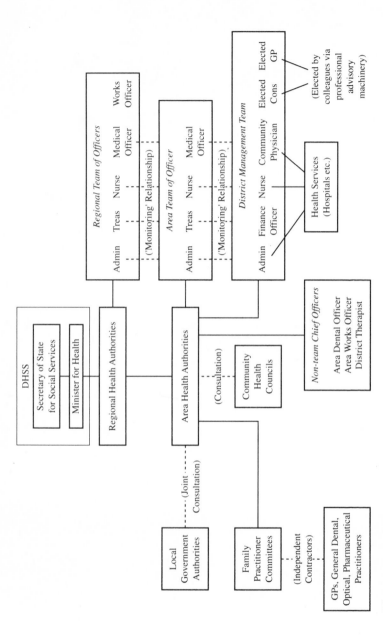

**Figure 3.1** Outline organization structure of English NHS; 1974

Although the new Conservative Government reiterated its continued commitment to consensus teams in *Patients First* (1979) and in its 1982 reorganization of the Service it was widely held that consensus teams reinforced the rather undynamic 'diplomat' model of management that we have already reviewed. Yet there was a crucial question which was rarely asked; was the system of consensus teams the *cause*, or the *consequence*, of 'diplomatic' management? The replacement of consensus management by general managers (the details of which we shall come to shortly) implied the former: abolish teams and management is strengthened. Yet, the alternative is perhaps more plausible: that the power of the health professionals in the 1970s was such that consensus teams were the only realistically available model for managing. It is easy to see that the view one adopts on this matter has important consequences for one's expectations of general managers. On the second view,

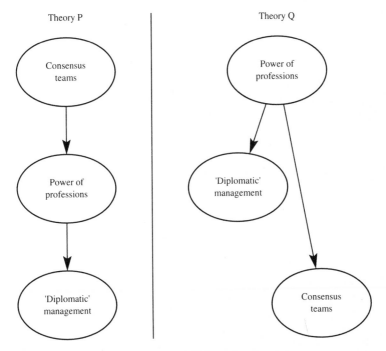

**Figure 3.2** Alternative theories of diplomatic management

abolishing consensus does little to change the underlying power relationships between professionals and managers. These alternative theories (for that is what they are) are summarized in Figure 3.2.

In October 1982 the (then) Mr Norman Fowler, Secretary of State for Social Services, announced at the Conservative Party Conference in October 1982 that he intended to establish a small team, headed by people from private industry, to ensure that 'manpower' was directed at serving the patient rather than building bureaucracy.

After initial difficulties in identifying a chairperson for this team, Mr Roy Griffiths, Deputy Chairman and Managing Director of the Sainsbury supermarket chain was invited to accept the role. After negotiating an extension to the terms of reference, so as to place emphasis on *management* rather than simply 'manpower', Mr Griffiths accepted. In February 1983, Mr Fowler announced (DHSS, Press Release no. 83/30, 3 February 1983) that:

> Four leading businessmen are to conduct an independent management Inquiry into the effective use and management of manpower and related resources in the National Health Service . . . we are setting the Inquiry two main tasks: to examine the way in which resources are used and controlled inside the health service, so as to secure the best value for money and the best possible services for the patient [and] to identify what further management issues need pursuing for these important purposes . . . Mr Griffiths has not been asked to prepare a report . . . we could simply have set up another Royal Commission and then sat back for several years to await its lengthy report, but on past experience that would not lead to effective action. Instead, we have gone straight for management action, with the minimum of fuss or formality.

The results of the team's deliberations were made public on 25 October 1983. We have summarized them using the clinical analogy of a diagnosis and prescription; this summary is set out in Table 3.2.[6]

If we look first at the 'diagnosis' column of Table 3.3, we can see how closely the four elements listed approximate to the four characteristics of the research-based picture of the 'diplomat' manager discussed earlier.

**Table 3.2**  The Griffiths diagnosis and prescription

| *The diagnosis* | *The prescription* |
| --- | --- |
| . . . it appears to us that consensus management can lead to 'lowest common denominator decisions' and to long delays in the management process . . . the absolute need to get agreement overshadows the substance of the decision required . . . In short, if Florence Nightingale were carrying her lamp through the corridors of the NHS today, she would almost certainly be searching for the people in charge (pp. 17, 22). | General managers in place of decision making by multi-professional consensus teams.<br><br>Establishment of general management in DHSS by separation of policy work from NHS management responsibilities. |
| . . . there is no driving force seeking and accepting direct and personal responsibility for developing management plans, securing their implementation and monitoring actual achievement . . . certain major initiatives are difficult to implement . . . [and] above all . . . lack of a general management process means that it is extremely difficult to achieve change . . . [A] more thrusting and committed style of management . . . is implicit in all our recommendations (pp. 12, 19). | Expansion of Regional review process.<br><br>Incentives and sanctions for individual managers. |
| Nor can the NHS display a ready assessment of the effectiveness with which it is meeting the needs and expectations of the people it serves. . . . Whether the NHS is meeting the needs of the patient, and the community, and can prove that it is doing so, is open to question (p. 10). | Consumer research.<br><br>More concern for consumer opinions. |
| . . . it lacks any real continuous evaluation of its performance . . . rarely are precise management objectives set; there is little measurement of health output; clinical evaluation of particular practices is by no means common and economic evaluation of these practices is extremely rare (p. 10). | Management budgets.<br><br>Cost-improvement programmes.<br><br>Continued use of performance indicators. |

*Source:* Quotations from NHS Management Inquiry, 1983. Crown copyright. Reproduced with the permission of Her Majesty's Stationery Office.

On 4 June 1984, Mr Fowler promulgated the Government's decisions on the Griffiths Report (DHSS Press Release no. 84/173, June 1984):

> . . . The Management Inquiry Team recommended that the general management function should be clearly vested in one person (at each level) who would take personal responsibility for securing action. We accept this view; and believe that the establishment of a personal and visible responsibility . . . is essential to obtain a guaranteed commitment . . . for improvement in services . . . In reaching this conclusion, we do not undervalue the importance of consensus in a multi-professional organisation like the NHS. But we share the Report's view that consensus, as a management style, will not alone secure effective and timely management action, nor does it necessarily initiate the kind of dynamic approach needed in the health service to ensure the best quality of care and value for money for patients.

General managers were therefore to be appointed at Regional, District and Unit levels of organization by the end of 1985; the posts were to be open to NHS managers of all disciplines, to doctors, and to persons from outside the Service. Appointments were to be on the basis of fixed-term contracts of three to five years with renewal for further fixed terms by mutual agreement and, by implication, dependent upon an assessment of the incumbent's performance. Any costs incurred by appointments were to be offset by savings on other management costs. More than 60 per cent of posts in the first round of appointments went to former administrators and treasurers. Only 12 per cent went to NHS 'outsiders', the largest single group amongst whom were not business people but military officers. Many of the doctors appointed were clinicians who undertook a part-time management role at unit level. Less than 10 per cent of posts went to nurses. More recent general manager appointments have been on rolling, rather than fixed-term contracts, and a system of individual performance review and performance-related pay has been introduced. The number of 'outsiders' appointed directly to general manager posts has fallen since the mid-1980s, as has the number of doctors in District and Unit general manager posts.

The post-Griffiths NHS, and the place of the general manager within it, is summarized in Figure 3.3. (Note that the DHSS was

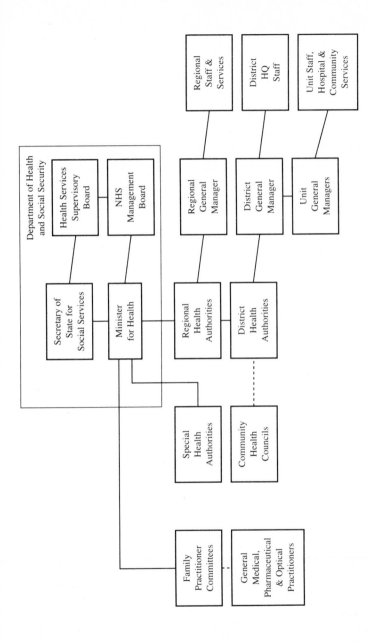

**Figure 3.3** Outline organizational structure of English NHS; 1987

*Source:* S. Harrison (1988) *Managing the National Health Service: Shifting the Frontier?* Chapman and Hall, London.

split into separate Departments of Health, and Social Security, in 1988.)

How far did the introduction of general managers constitute an effective challenge to professional groups? In place of consensus decision-making teams (with a heavy professional membership), and other professional heads responsible directly to their employing Authorities, were individual general managers, with ostensible authority over all staff employed within their Region, Unit or District. On the other hand research carried out in the wake of the Griffiths changes suggests that while general managers were frequently successful in asserting control over nurses and the professions supplementary to medicine, their impact on medical autonomy was much less marked.[7] Hence we discuss the two groups separately.

First, the non-medical professionals: one of the general managers first tasks was, of course, to devise an organization structure for the area of their authority, and this put the question of the single-professional management hierarchies (especially nursing) on their agenda from the beginning. This necessity, coupled with the very considerable freedom which was accorded to general managers in respect of local organization structure gave them a great deal of immediate power over nurses and the paramedical professions, since organization structures are a prime source of organizational rewards (they largely determine gradings, and hence salaries). General managers were able both to create new, non-professionally defined, roles, and to sideline or dispose of staff whom they did not see as fitting into the new requirements for managing the NHS. Box 3.1 sets out some vivid quotations from respondents to one post-Griffiths research study.

In addition to changing management hierarchies, general managers were also able to open up questions of professional roles and skill mix: to ask, for instance, whether many nursing activities really required trained staff, or whether much health visitor work might not be more appropriately performed by a social worker.

Yet despite this, and despite the widespread, if grudging, acceptance of general managers by nurses (after an initial campaign against Griffiths) and paramedical professionals, there is evidence of an 'implementation gap'. The experience of many NHS employees in the years immediately after Griffiths was of lots of top management pronouncements and 'initiatives' but little of substance at the level of delivery of services to patients. This was

---

**Box 3.1** Nursing and general management

- 'There's always been an opportunity to get rid of poor quality staff in the NHS but we've never taken advantage of it.' (Unit general manager; p. 69.)
- 'We've got to pick winners. We've picked three good people out of the woodwork at St. Luke's. The [nursing] hierarchy stopped them in the past.' (District general manager; p. 72.)
- 'The previous [District Nursing Officer] was very much an autocrat . . . and for her the nurses were always right. She was very much a tribalist . . . I'm very sceptical of some modern nursing claims; the idea that we can claim monopoly rights on care.' (Chief Nursing Adviser; p. 73.)
- '[The nursing role in giving professional advice is] Bloody unintelligible! It's all they've got to hang on to. It's a load of cobblers in terms of corporate advice [to health authorities.] If you want professional advice from nurses – say if you need to build a new hospital . . . you can get it just for that particular job. To pay £25 000 a year for it is a disgrace. Professional advice is a load of hogwash! The only justification for them in management team positions has been the power of the profession.' (Regional general manager; p. 98.)

*Source:* P. Strong and J. Robinson (1990) *The NHS Under New Management.* Open University Press, Milton Keynes.

---

perhaps particularly the case in the area of 'consumerism'. Nevertheless, the overall conclusion must be that general managers had substantially more control over non-medical health professionals than had their administrative predecessors.

What, then, about general managers and doctors? It is clear that in one specific area, additional powers of control were acquired by general managers; it became much easier than it had been for administrators to close hospital beds and to make other changes in services without extended periods of consultation. But, in the early years of the Griffiths changes, this was the sole substantial difference between the ability of general managers to control doctors, and that of their predecessors. In other areas of organizational life, doctors retained virtually undiminished their ability to obstruct changes of which they disapproved. Indeed in some research they tended to report that the Griffiths changes had not decreased their influence. Moreover, it seems that doctors retained a good deal of *covert* influence; many general managers expected doctors to be difficult, and therefore refrained from raising issues that might arouse opposition, preferring instead to leave matters to be dealt with by peer pressure. Younger hospital consultants were sometimes, however, reported as being more pliant.

How can we explain these research findings? Why were general managers not more influential with doctors? A large part of the answer lies in the financial context of the NHS at the time of the introduction of the Griffiths changes. The research shows that general managers' personal agendas were dominated by two considerations: the need to implement the changes themselves, and the need to ensure that their organizations remained within tight financial constraints. Not surprisingly, therefore, general managers tended to concentrate on achieving these crucial objectives (which, of course, might well entail closing beds and making other service changes), and otherwise on changes which were most easily achievable, such as those in formal organization structure. In addition, symbolic 'initiatives' would help to maintain the external impression of more substantially pro-active managerial activity. This pressing external agenda was by no means the only source of managerial weakness. Many general managers regarded their fixed-term appointments as another.

Despite the rhetoric of the time, therefore, there was little that could be regarded as the major shift in NHS 'culture' that many of the proponents of Griffiths had called for. The 'diplomatic' approach to management was still practised, especially in relation to doctors. But, perhaps oddly, the research showed that general managers had one attribute that, as it transpired would be a necessary, though not sufficient, element in later attempts to control professionals through the introduction of a market in health care (see Chapter 5). This attribute was credibility; despite all the evidence about modest substantive impact, people found the NHS under general managers a less frustrating place to work than it had been under consensus teams.

With hindsight, the introduction of general management can be seen to have had one more further significant consequence. It put in place a spine of generalists, working on performance-related contracts and subject to hierarchical instruction from the NHS management board down. Having this cadre in place was to provide the Government with a powerful tool for implementation when, in 1989, the most major reform was announced.

## MANAGEMENT INFORMATION

In most textbook definitions of management, the functions of allocating resources and measuring performance are seen as central tasks. For rational decision-making about either, task relevant information is obviously crucial. One way in which burgeoning NHS managers could challenge professionals was therefore to confront the latter with telling new performance information. Indeed, this was frequently attempted. To understand, however, why it was not (and still is not) an entirely straightforward strategy we need to understand some very general points about the 'politics of information'.

An organization of any size performs an infinite variety of activities, and it is literally impossible for managers directly to supervise all of these, for at least two reasons. One is obvious: there is insufficient time, and managerial time must be rationed in some way. Slightly less obviously, it is simply not possible for managers fully to understand everything that happens within an organization.[8] However extensive their training and however relevant their personal expertise, they cannot have performed every job in the organization. This means that they cannot know how to *value* many of the organization's activities.

One way in which managers cope with such problems is by constructing management information systems. Such systems embody a prior judgement, implicit or explicit, about which activities it is most important to control; this determines the information items collected by the system. Thus the system, once created, automatically apportions at least part of the manager's time. (To the extent that information systems are often designed by outside agencies, such as management consultants, or by middle level technical staff, top managers are therefore allowing themselves to be controlled from elsewhere!)

Choosing information items, however, does not solve the whole of the manager's problem. There is a further problem of how to

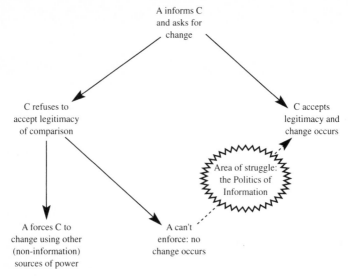

**Figure 3.4**    The power of management information? (Assume that A has information that B's performance is better than C's)

'read' the information provided by the system. What is 'good' and what is 'bad'? One way of answering (or sometimes avoiding!) this question is to set targets, standards or norms. For instance, managers may determine a target ratio of $x$ whole-time equivalent nurses to $y$ hospital beds. This approach can have drawbacks especially if a plethora of absolute targets are set in the face of the many uncertainties in the contemporary organizational environment. If such absolute approaches are abandoned, or judged suitable in only a few circumstances, it is necessary to turn to relativist ones, that is, to employ *comparisons*. Such comparisons can examine differences over time within one organization, or differences between (comparable) organizations at a particular point in time, or both. As we shall see shortly, management information systems in the NHS developed along these relativist lines during the 1980s and early 1990s.

Before we turn to the specifics of the NHS, however, we need to examine the further conditions which would have to be met if management information were to play any part in imposing managerial will upon professionals. 'Information is power' runs the cliché, but we believe this to be a considerable oversimplification.

...s the case. Our analysis is illustrated

by
com
terms
If C *do*
recogni.
accurate,
ance). Suc
A's values
*suasion*, not
'conditioned'
legitimacy of t.
because he or sh
ted with informal
can be compelled.

'better' than C's, and that A
C may or may not respond in
the direction desired by A.
two reasons. First, C may
on (that is, that it is
assessing perform-

If C *does not* in_ually respond to A's communication of the information by changing behaviour, A may enforce the change by using other sources of power. If A is unable to do so, it may be because such other sources are inadequate or because C is able to mount a successful challenge on the legitimacy of the comparison.

All this suggests that *of itself*, performance information of the type described is only a source of power where its legitimacy is recognized by those over whom the power is exercised (the Bs and Cs). From the point of view of those who seek to exercise power (the As), a preferred strategy may well be to seek prior acceptance by the B's and C's of A's chosen criteria of performance; then the use of performance information can become unobtrusive and largely self-regulating. It may therefore be hypothesized that the 'politics of management information' will focus on a struggle to impose legitimacy upon a particular set of comparisons.

More specifically, it may be expected that the As will: (i) seek to establish a consensual basis for the comparison of the performance of Bs and Cs, using strategies such as working groups and creating a style of rhetoric consonant with the chosen basis of performance; (ii) seek to establish information systems and specifications which are standardized in the way in which they relate to those over whom control is sought; (iii) seek to identify a small number of key measures of performance. In contrast, it may be expected that Bs and Cs (etc.) will (iv) seek to avoid the standardization of information systems and specifications; and, wherever they know, or fear, that their performance is relatively poor in respect to A's criteria, (v) seek to establish alternative and additional criteria, undermine A's criteria, point to trade-offs between alternative measures, and so on. Finally, in those cases where (vi) A has established criteria which appear to show the performance of B or C in a *favourable* light, B or C may be prepared to use this information to bolster their reputation or bid for more resources yet still reserve the right to criticize the criteria in future, if and when their application produces less flattering 'results'.

The story of NHS 'performance indicators' begins with the Comptroller and Auditor-General, the statutory auditor of government expenditure, now head of the National Audit Office who had for some years taken an increasing interest in value-for-money audit as opposed to narrow financial propriety. In his annual report on the Appropriation Accounts for 1979–80, wide discrepancies in staffing levels were noted between health authorities. As quoted in the Committee of Public Accounts, Seventh Report (1981: 1) these observations raised

> . . . the question of the right balance, in the interests of economy and efficiency, between the necessary central direction and oversight of the NHS and a system of delegation and discretion appropriate to a locally-based and managed service.

The Public Accounts Committee (PAC), to whom the Comptroller's reports are rendered, took up this matter in a series of hearings in the spring of 1981. Throughout these, members of the Committee stressed the NHS's accountability to Parliament and emphasized their perceptions of a lack of Department of Health and Social Security (DHSS) control over health authorities.

The response of DHSS witnesses was to argue that detailed central control was unnecessary; the system of cash limits and promulgation of central government priorities meant that it was appropriate for health authorities to develop localized approaches. In their Report, the Committee reached a compromise conclusion; there should be no detailed central control, but instead a greater upward flow of information as a means of monitoring the comparative performance of health authorities (ibid.: xvii):

> . . . arrangements will be satisfactory in practice only if accountability upwards is matched by a flow of information about the activities of the districts, which will enable the regions, and

in turn DHSS, to monitor performance effectively and to take necessary action to remedy any serious deficiencies, or inefficiency, which may develop.

These critical remarks were amongst the first problems to be faced by the new Secretary of State, Mr Norman Fowler, who assumed office in mid-1981. The solution was announced by him in January 1982: Performance Indicators were to be developed on a pilot basis in the Northern Region.[9] To be employed in conjunction with the review process. They would (DHSS, Press Release No. 82/14 1982: 2):

> . . . enable comparison to be made between districts and so help Ministers and the Regional Chairmen . . . to assess the performance of their constituent . . . authorities in using manpower and other resources efficiently.

The first national package of indicators was issued in September 1983. It was in a form which allowed any health authority to be compared with all others in terms both of absolute values of the indicators used and of rankings within the region and the country. The package contained some 70 indicators relating to clinical work, finance, 'manpower', support services and estate management, all constructed from already available data. The clinical indicators related mainly to the use of clinical facilities within broad specialty groups, rather than to the outcomes of treatment. They consisted primarily of efficiency measures as average length of hospital stay, throughput of patients per bed, intervals between cases occupying a bed, and the ratio of return outpatient visits to new outpatients. Notice that these are all measures which are largely determined by the aggregate of doctors' behaviour rather than by managers' decisions.

A number of criticisms were made of the first indicator package. First, indicators were ambiguous in that it was not clear whether high, or low, values represented 'good' performance. Second, it was known that many of the original data sources were of dubious accuracy. Third, the physical format of indicator presentation in a very thick book of typescript tables was held to be user-unfriendly. Finally, the absence of data related to health care outcome was criticized. A number of joint DHSS/NHS working groups were established to revise the indicators, and to extend them beyond hospitals, and a revised package was issued in July 1985. The new indicators went some way towards meeting the second and third criticisms (in particular, by using computer graphics), but still lacked measures related to the effectiveness of treatment. An indicator of medically preventable deaths was added in 1987.[10]

Various modifications have been made both to the content and presentation of indicators, which cover a broad range of hospital activity and some community activity (including acute, elderly, children's, mental illness, mental handicap and support services) as well as 'manpower', which of course reflects their origins in the concerns of the PAC. Despite many improvements, however, a recent survey of the use of indicators by different types of organization concluded that (Carter 1992: 169):

> while our studies showed that nearly all organisations were beginning to move . . . towards the prescriptive use of indicators, i.e. setting objectives and targets against which performance can be measured – the NHS and the police remain behind the pack.

It may be helpful to look at an actual example of NHS performance indicator data. Table 3.3 represents some of the general surgical indicators for the districts in the Yorkshire NHS region, together with regional and national averages. Each double column is headed by the code number of the indicator which it represents, the short titles of the indicators (note, *not* the definitions) being given alongside their respective codes at the bottom.

Within each double column, there are two figures given. The left-hand one (headed 'value') is the numerical value of the actual indicator; different indicators are in different units. In this example, columns 1, 2 and 4 are in days, and column 3 is a percentage, and column 5 is deaths/discharges per bed. The right-hand one (headed 'per cent rank') shows percentile ranking, which shows the location of a particular District on a particular indicator, relative to the rest of England. Hence, in this example Scarborough is in the top 4 per cent of the country on length of stay for surgery, whilst Leeds Western is in the bottom 6 per cent. *'Top' and 'bottom' are expressed solely in numerical terms.* Thus, if you assume (which is not self-evident, as is argued below) that efficient bed usage is important, then you will want (like Scarborough) to be at the numerical top on indicator A10A, but at the numerical bottom on A24A. A number of the Performance Indicators (PIs) themselves have been standardized in an attempt to ensure that meaningful

**Table 3.3** DHSS Performance Indicators for 1985/86 General surgical 1st line PIs. Table 5 of 8 indicators (see text)

| Area | A10A* | | A10B | | A10C | | A17 | | A21A | |
|---|---|---|---|---|---|---|---|---|---|---|
| | value | per cent rank | value | per cent rank | value | per cent rank | value | per cent rank | value | per cent rank |
| Hull | 7.80 | 81 | 7.80 | 97 | 100. | 55 | 2.90 | 89 | 34.1 | 10 |
| E. Yorkshire | 6.10 | 23 | 5.80 | 2 | 105. | 66 | 6.90 | 100 | 28.1 | 1 |
| Grimsby | 6.70 | 43 | 6.40 | 12 | 105. | 66 | 3.20 | 93 | 36.9 | 22 |
| Scunthorpe | 6.20 | 28 | 6.60 | 23 | 94.0 | 34 | 2.30 | 71 | 42.9 | 62 |
| Northallerton | 7.50 | 73 | 7.00 | 60 | 107. | 70 | 2.80 | 87 | 35.4 | 15 |
| York | 6.60 | 40 | 6.80 | 42 | 97.0 | 46 | 3.10 | 92 | 37.6 | 26 |
| Scarborough | 5.20 | 4 | 7.10 | 67 | 73.0 | 1 | .600 | 2 | 62.9 | 99 |
| Harrogate | 7.60 | 75 | 6.40 | 12 | 119. | 90 | 2.80 | 87 | 35.1 | 13 |
| Bradford | 7.10 | 61 | 6.40 | 12 | 111. | 80 | 2.70 | 83 | 37.2 | 25 |
| Airedale | 7.40 | 71 | 6.80 | 42 | 109. | 76 | 2.80 | 87 | 35.8 | 16 |
| Calderdale | 8.20 | 87 | 6.70 | 31 | 122. | 93 | 2.90 | 89 | 32.9 | 5 |
| Huddersfield | 6.10 | 23 | 6.30 | 9 | 97.0 | 46 | 3.50 | 96 | 38.0 | 29 |
| Dewsbury | 6.10 | 23 | 6.40 | 12 | 95.0 | 37 | 1.20 | 15 | 50.0 | 90 |
| Leeds Western | 9.00 | 95 | 7.20 | 75 | 125. | 94 | 1.60 | 35 | 34.4 | 11 |
| Leeds Eastern | 8.40 | 91 | 7.00 | 60 | 120. | 91 | .900 | 7 | 39.2 | 40 |
| Wakefield | 6.80 | 47 | 6.70 | 31 | 101. | 59 | 3.10 | 92 | 36.9 | 22 |
| Pontefract | 6.90 | 50 | 6.90 | 53 | 100. | 55 | 2.50 | 77 | 38.8 | 37 |
| | | | | | | | | | | |
| Yorkshire | 7.20 | | 6.80 | | 106. | | 2.40 | | 38.0 | |
| | | | | | | | | | | |
| England | 6.90 | | 6.90 | | 100. | | 1.90 | | 41.5 | |
| no. DHAs | | 191 | | 191 | | 191 | | 191 | | 191 |

* A10A, Actual length of stay-general surgery (GS); A10B, expected length of stay-GS; A10C, standardized LoS ratio-GS; A17, turnover interval-GS; A24A, actual throughput-GS.

*Source:* Crown copyright. Reproduced with the permission of Her Majesty's Stationery Office.

comparisons are made. Consider the following example; Table 3.3 shows that Leeds Western's *actual throughput* (A24A) is 34.4 (patients per bed, per annum). But Leeds Western's patients differ from the national average in terms of both age/sex ratios and diagnostic mix within the specialty, and hence an *expected throughput* (A24B) can be calculated by applying this mix to national rates of activity. This gives a figure of 40.1, presumably reflecting a tendency to treat younger and/or less sick patients (defined by ICD category) than the country in general. Finally, *standardized throughput* (A24C) can be expressed by taking actual as a percentage of expected; in the case of Leeds Western 34.4 as a percentage of 40.1 is 80 per cent. A figure of 100 per cent would thus mean a District or Unit was performing 'as expected' on a particular indicator.

These, then are the technical aspects of performance indicators.[11] What are their implications for the control of health professionals? Although not *all* the several hundred indicators in use measure the work of professionals directly, a very large number do. A glance at Table 3.3 and back at our discussion of pre-Griffiths research findings at the beginning of this chapter will reinforce the point. And two of the three hypotheses that we proposed earlier in this section concerning A's behaviour are indeed borne out. PIs are in a standardized format, so as to facilitate comparison, and their development has largely been achieved through the use of consensual working parties rather than through political or managerial diktat. Management certainly has *not* been able to focus the exercise on a few key indicators, or to attach clear operational targets to these. On the contrary, the total number of PIs grew and grew, until, as we go to press, there was a further attempt to produce a few, key, indicators (*The Times*, 2 March 1993: 2).

Meanwhile the professionals (the 'B's and 'C's in terms of Figure 3.4) have certainly acted as if they feared that their performance would appear poor, by seeking to undermine the legitimacy of the criteria implied by PIs in several of the ways that we suggested. Many criticisms of the use of PIs have been made, e.g.:

● There is a temptation for managers to put things right by taking action to change the numerical value of the indicator whilst ignoring the underlying problem. For example, there is the practice of many health authorities in counting a discharge when a patient is transferred to another hospital.

**Box 3.2**   What are PIs and what are they for?

PIs are statistical information which enable you to compare the performance of your service with that achieved by others. They are calculated from data which have been available for many years but were of limited value until now because they have not been presented in ways relevant to your needs as a manager. PIs present the information in a systematic, consistent and helpful way, making it possible to compare the performance of services in different hospitals and districts.

PIs are intended to stimulate a *spirit of enquiry*. Being accountable for a service you will be concerned not only about how that service appears to be performing from a local viewpoint, but also how it is performing in comparison with services elsewhere and, eventually, over time. With PIs you can compare the performance of districts or hospitals in your region or throughout England.

PIs are indicators not measures. Health services are too complex, and measuring their end product too difficult, to permit exact and comprehensive measurement of performance – at least on the basis of our present knowledge. PIs will help you to identify aspects of service which *may* need further investigation. You should not take action solely on the basis of PIs. Rather you should look at other information available to you locally and then discuss the position with colleagues involved in providing the service. Only then should you make a decision about whether any action needs to be taken; that decision will ultimately be based on your own professional judgement.

*Source:* Department of Health and Social Security (1986) *Performance Indicators for the NHS: Guidance for Users*. DHSS, London. Crown copyright. Reproduced with the permission of Her Majesty's Stationery Office.

- The focus on 'outliers' (extreme scores) in the ranking means that managers may not stop to look at what indicators mean, despite the plethora of official disclaimers, such as that set out in Box 3.2.
- The focus on outliers also tends to lead to the assumption that if

one is not an outlier there is no problem; this is not necessarily or even probably the case.

- As noted already, the PIs and the format in which they are presented, deal only in high and low *numerical* values. Consequently, what is 'good' and 'bad' remains a matter of interpretation.
- Given the large number of indicators, it is almost certain that a manager will find himself/herself confronted with a pattern of 'good' performance on some PIs, and 'poor' to others. This raises not only difficulties of interpretation (which careful study of advice given in the manuals and/or the use of an expert system can resolve) but the possibility that action taken to improve one PI will worsen another. The most obvious examples relate to bed usage; all other things equal, reducing length of stay will increase turnover interval for instance.

In the face of these difficulties, it is hardly surprising that PIs are still rarely seen as legitimate in professional circles within the NHS. In order to use them as control mechanisms, therefore, managers would have to resort to other sources of power or influence.

So far as possible, managers seem to have avoided this; in practice, PIs have mainly been used as a currency of discussion between the DHSS/Department of Health (DoH),[12] Regions, and District Health Authorities, that is, between different levels of manager, rather than between managers and professionals. In general, therefore, PIs have been used in a reactive, rather than strategic, fashion: as a buttress to an established policy stance rather than as an aid to reaching a new one. Moreover, there is research to suggest not only that many managers were unable fully to understand the potential significance of complex arrays of indicator values, but that many feared the ability of professionals to 'turn the argument around' and use the figures to demand additional resources.[13]

Our conclusion is, therefore, that the type of management information characterized by NHS performance indicators has not had a systematic impact on health professionals, though it is certainly the case that some of the latter will have found themselves on the receiving end of pressure to move away from the extremes of the rankings. Such systems require either to be assimilated into professional culture (i.e. become seen as professionally legitimate) or to be backed by stronger incentives and sanctions than were available to NHS managers during the 1980s.

## CHALLENGING THE UNIONS

The two challenges to professional autonomy we have just examined both involved the creation of some kind of countervailing influence – in the first instance general management and in the second a new framework of performance information which was intended for use by senior management to tighten the latter's grip on how the professional groups were carrying out their activities. In this final section we look at an even more direct challenge: not the creation of a countervailing influence but a direct attempt to reduce the power and independence of those organizations which represented the NHS work force.

Much of this third challenge was centrally driven, with local managements varying considerably in their degree of enthusiasm or reservation about the Government's reforms. Behind the details of these reforms one can discern the gradual and partial emergence of the new model of management referred to in the final section of Chapter 1. The old model – a rough and ready consensus which had survived from 1945 until the late 1970s – comprised Government support for the principle of collective bargaining, for the (national, centralized) Whitley system and for an essentially voluntarist framework of trade union law. The new model, by contrast, bears the marks of its 'new right' or neo-liberal origins. The stress is on individualism, the healthiness of market forces and the need for legal curbs on the powers of trade unions, especially in the area of strikes and disputes. National agreements are regarded as often rigid and restrictive, and local management flexibility to hire, fire and set pay and conditions is favoured instead. Professional groups, however, may escape some of the rigours of this tougher approach, but usually only if they have been prepared to offer the Government some quid pro quo in the shape of, for example, a no-strike agreement and/or a commitment to salary restraint. If they do offer up some much self-denying ordnance then they may be rewarded with their own special machinery for settling pay and conditions.

One further conceptual preliminary needs to be explained. We have chosen to structure our account by employing Alan Fox's distinction between 'market relations' and 'managerial relations' (Fox 1966: 6):

> Market relations have to do with the terms and conditions on which labour is hired – they are therefore economic in

character. Managerial relations arise out of what management seeks to do with its labour having hired it. They have to do with the exercise of authority and can for this reason be termed political in character.

Of course, these categories are not mutually exclusive; for example, decisions about working hours (managerial relations) may well have an impact on pay (market relations). Nevertheless, the distinction is a useful one for our purposes. We begin with market relations, and, as in previous sections with a brief look at history.[14]

From the early 1970s, the trades unions with members in the NHS were increasingly seen as flexing their muscles. For a number of the unions operating in the NHS its employees provided the last large pool of unorganized labour covered by their constitutions, and by 1972 the spread (with management agreement) of the 'check off' from salaries of union subscriptions meant that membership could be retained more easily, and heightened the necessity for competitive recruitment. From the management side, there has never been active discouragement of union membership of the kind found in industry, and it is plausible to suppose that the replacement of paternalism by managerialism would have removed a psychological barrier to membership. In particular, the introduction of bonus schemes from about 1968 onwards meant that *local* management–union discussions had to take place, endowing local union activity with legitimacy.

By the mid-1970s, these changes had coalesced into industrial relations behaviour which was both more localized and more conflictual than before. Increasing local activism was the result both of the intentions of unions such as the National Union of Public Employees and the Transport and General Workers Union to decentralize, and of management's need to negotiate incentive schemes and the kind of procedure agreements recommended by the codes of practice issued under post-1971 employment legislation. Local stewards were legitimized by national Whitley agreements of 1971 and 1976, and many joint consultative committees were established or revived during this period.

Many health professionals, especially nurses, were members of traditional unions, such as those mentioned above, or the Confederation of Health Service Employees. Others, however, were members of what were generally referred to as 'professional associations': the Royal College of Nursing (RCN) and Midwifery, the Society of Radiographers, and so on. (Some, though it was never known how many, were members of both types of organization.) These latter organizations had a collective bargaining role just as the more traditional unions did, and possessed seats on the 'staff sides' of the Whitley Councils, the joint government department/NHS employing authority/union bodies responsible for negotiating salaries and terms and conditions of employment of NHS staff.

Not unnaturally, the professional associations felt the need to respond to the growth of the other unions, and most transformed themselves into legally defined trade unions during the mid-1970s. Along with this change went others: the introduction of the check-off (probably the main cause of massive RCN membership growth between 1977 and 1980), the appointment of local stewards (in the case of the smaller professional unions, on a joint basis), and an increasing acquiescence in militancy.

Associated with these changes was the markedly greater degree of industrial action which occurred within the NHS after 1972. Prior to this time, such action had been rare (though not unknown), and the 1972–73 ancillary staff industrial action in support of a national pay claim represented a break with the past both in terms of its scale and its readiness to include strike action. The remainder of the 1970s saw a high level of various kinds of industrial action by virtually all groups of NHS staff, though strikes were generally less significant than other forms of coercive action such as overtime bans, working to rule, and the provision of emergency services only. Also a number of 'work-ins' occurred at hospitals scheduled for closure. The culmination was the 'winter of discontent' of 1978–79, which may well have played a part in the Labour Government's defeat at the polls in May 1979.

Despite this increase in union activity across almost all classes of NHS employee, the results were not encouraging from a union point of view. Major disputes did not result in significantly increased management offers. One, quite widespread, perception of this on the union side was that lack of unity between different staff groups was an important contributory factor. Helped by the movement of the annual pay settlement date for ancillary staff to 1 April, the same as that for other staff groups, the next major dispute, in 1982, saw an unprecedented degree of cooperation and coordination between the different kinds of union and different NHS staff groups, though this is not to suggest that there were not also tensions.[15]

Although the dispute was ended without substantial movement in the Government's offer, the apparently emergent inter-group and inter-union solidarity which had been manifested was sufficient of a threat for the Government to seek to disrupt it. The chosen vehicle was a Pay Review Body for nurses, midwives and certain other health professions who wished to participate. The Review Body was along the lines established for the medical profession as long ago as the 1950s: the replacement of *pay* negotiations (other conditions of service would continue to be negotiated) with an independent body to which the parties, including the unions and health authorities, could submit evidence. The Review Body would make recommendations to the Prime Minister, who could accept them in whole or in part.

Following discussions with the professions, the new Review Body for Nursing Staff, Midwives, Health Visitors and Professions Allied to Medicine was announced in January 1983.[16] The creation of this body disrupted potential union solidarity in two ways. First, it was selective; neither non-professional groups (such as the ancillaries) nor professional groups with a preponderance of members in the traditional unions (such as laboratory scientific staff) were offered participation. (Speech therapists declined to participate.) Second, though no consequences ever flowed from this statement, participation was to be confined to groups who did not take industrial action. This wedge between those covered and those not covered was subsequently driven deeper by the consistent awards of more favourable pay increases to the former group than to the latter.

It seems clear, however, that the creation of the Review Body can best be seen as an opportunistic device for challenging the unions rather than as a policy commitment to a particular model of NHS labour relations. Not only were subsequent requests (by groups such as speech therapists and general managers) to be included in the ambit of the Review Body refused, but the whole future of national pay determination, of which the latter was a part, began to be placed in doubt. Since 1983, there had been a slowly growing body of opinion amongst health authorities and NHS managers that greater local flexibility in pay determination was desirable.

The arguments underpinning this view were varied,[17] but its gradual acceptance within the NHS has been one of the crucial prerequisites for the acceptance of the decentralized labour relations role of the NHS Trusts created by the Government's 1989 NHS reforms. We shall be discussing Trusts more fully in Chapter 5. It is sufficient in this chapter to note that they are not bound by Whitley Council or other central terms and conditions of employment, except in so far as existing staff at the date of Trust creation are entitled to retain their existing contractual arrangement. Although, at present, Trusts have not moved sharply away from national agreements, there is evidence that such moves have at least been contemplated. Moreover, most Trusts so far established seem to be planning restrictions in their recognition of unions.[18]

It has perhaps also contributed to a growing perception amongst health authorities and managers that the existence of extensive formalized staff appeals mechanisms is no longer desirable. The more immediate cause of the Secretary of State for Health's unilateral decision in 1992 to discontinue the regional and national grievance and grading appeals procedures was the immense backlog of appeals against the outcomes of the new nurses' clinical grading structure introduced in 1988. It seems likely, however, that if one nationally negotiated agreement can be unilaterally abandoned, others can too. The effect of such a change is disrupt potential union solidarity along a second dimension: that of geography.

Indeed, other unilateral changes were made: a new contract for GPs was introduced in 1990 without the agreement of the profession. Quite apart from the manner of its introduction, its use of 'target payments' for cervical cytology and for vaccination/immunization is a good indication of the use of market relations for policy purposes, i.e. to affect managerial relations.

In summary, then, it seems that the position of health professionals in market relations has been substantially weakened in the last decade. As we have seen, the Government challenge to the professional unions has resulted in cleavage of the incipient union solidarity of 1982 along two dimensions. First, the occupational dimension: professionals have been detached from other categories of worker. Second, the geographical dimension: there is a move towards fragmenting the pay determination even within an occupation. Of course, it is not possible to assess the consequences of these changes in terms of pay awards; we cannot know what would otherwise have occurred. But the intent has been clear, given the importance of labour costs as approximately 70 per cent of NHS revenue expenditure.

It is not only *rates* of pay that determine the costs of a workforce.

The way in which it is trained, demarcated, and controlled will also be important determinants. These matters are the stuff of what we referred to above as 'managerial relations', to which we now turn. The topic is a large one, so that we are able here to do no more than illustrate the increasing control over health professionals in three areas: career opportunities, staffing levels and the demarcation of duties.

First, we consider nursing careers, where the effect of the Griffiths changes has been the loss of the right to be managed exclusively by a member of the same profession, a right which was consolidated in the 1974 structure of the NHS. This amounts to the loss of guaranteed promotion opportunities, and it is hardly surprising that the reaction of the nursing unions to the Griffiths general management proposals was hostile.

The views of the Royal College of Nursing, the Royal College of Midwives, the Association of Nurse Administrators, the Confederation of Health Service Employees, and the National Union of Public Employees were highly consistent. They expressed concern at the short consultation period, at the absence of the (then) Department of Health and Social Security chief nursing officer from the proposed management board, and at the absence of a trial period for the new management arrangements. They also indicated a general desire to retain consensus decision-making (though the Royal College of Nursing was prepared to give up the veto power of each team member), and to retain a line relationship between district nursing officer and directors of nursing services within units. These organizations also resisted the idea of nursing budgets being held by non-nurses and the potential for a general manager to compel a nurse to 'act unprofessionally'. In general, there was a feeling that Griffiths had paid scant regard to the status or professionalism of nurses, a notion subsequently carried by the Royal College of Nursing into an anti-Griffiths national advertising campaign.

These concerns about the Griffiths proposals produced, on the face of it, a number of concessions on the part of the Government. The Department's chief nursing officer was included in the NHS Management Board, and although English districts were not required to retain district nursing officers (as the profession's representatives had hoped), they were required by the Secretary of State to provide for a senior officer to give nursing advice to the authority (in Wales and Scotland, chief nursing officers were retained at health authority level).

**Table 3.4**   The background of NHS general managers

| Former occupation | RGM | | DGM | | UGM | | Percentage of all | |
|---|---|---|---|---|---|---|---|---|
| | *1986* | *1987* | *1986* | *1987* | *1986* | *1987* | *1986* | *1987* |
| NHS admin. and finance | 9 | 9 | 132 | 132 | 364 | 355 | 62 | 61 |
| NHS medicine | 1 | 1 | 15 | 16 | 110 | 110 | 15 | 16 |
| NHS nursing | 1 | 1 | 4 | 5 | 70 | 71 | 9 | 9 |
| NHS other | – | – | – | – | – | 14 | – | 2 |
| Outside NHS | 3 | 3 | 38 | 36 | 54 | 57 | 12 | 12 |
| Vacancies | – | – | 2 | 2 | 13 | 4 | 2 | 1 |
| Total | 14 | 14 | 191 | 191 | 611 | 611 | | ** |

\* *Abbreviations:*
RGM Regional General Manager; DGM District General Manager; UGM Unit General Manager.
\*\* Percentages do not necessarily sum to 100 due to rounding.

*Sources:*
October 1986. S. Harrison (1988) *Managing the National Health Service: Shifting the Frontier?*, 66. Chapman and Hall, London.
December 1987. A. Leathard (1990) *Health Care Provision: Past, Present and Future*, 89. Chapman and Hall, London.

Nevertheless, it is difficult not to interpret the outcome as an important defeat for the nursing unions, both traditional and professional. The impact upon nurses is to some extent indicated by their relatively low rate of success in obtaining General Manager posts. As Table 3.4 shows, they fared worse than any other group in the initial round of post-Griffiths appointments, a position not significantly improved upon by the end of 1987.

Nurses were, however, quick to capitalize upon Griffiths' emphasis on the impact of health care upon the patient, and the report's implementation period has seen a gradual acceptance of a reorientation of nurse management towards this. Many senior nurses have been appointed to posts concerned with such work – such as director of quality assurance – and it is possible thereby that nurse managers' overall career opportunities will be no worse than before Griffiths.

We now turn to the management control of staffing levels in nursing, an area in which there has been a degree of interest since at least the 1970s, when systems began to develop based on a variety of factors, from patient dependence to the results of systematic consultation amongst nurse managers.[19] More recent developments have, however, both included the notion of quality and taken a much more industrial approach towards staffing levels. The North American GRASP system, for instance, employs what is in effect time-study data concerning individual nursing tasks and aggregates it into a staffing requirement.

This system is currently being introduced into a number of UK hospitals. The 'Monitor' system (a derivative of another North American system) concerns itself with quality of nursing care, something which earlier methods had tended to take for granted, and seems to be being quite widely implemented in the NHS. Taken in the context of a critical 1985 report by the Comptroller and Auditor General and the Public Accounts Committee's subsequent interest in the topic, these kinds of developments, if introduced widely, would offer much greater managerial control over nurses than is presently exercised.[20] Yet, unlike the other developments directly associated with Griffiths, they have apparently given rise to very little disapproval within the profession, although they have been quite widely discussed in the nursing press. This is perhaps because they are seen as mere technicalities by rank-and-file nurses while, for nurse managers, responsibility for the implementation and oversight of such systems may compensate for status lost in the Griffiths changes. For ward sisters, charge nurses, and rank-and-file nurses, on the other hand, the impact may well be different, since it is upon them that the weight of new systems of control will fall. There has been no parallel attempt to control medical staffing levels.[21] Indeed, the great difficulty in this area has been in *increasing* the numbers of consultant medical staff in relation to their juniors; to a great extent the former group has successfully avoided the additional 'on-call' commitment and routine ('less interesting') work which would follow from such a change.[22]

Finally, we turn to the changing rules of work demarcation between occupations in the NHS. Such changes, of course, have been a feature of UK health services since before the inception of the NHS; for instance, sections of the medical profession sought to retain direct control over radiographic work from the turn of the century until about 1920. Indeed, the general pattern of such changes in the division of labour has taken the form of the transfer of work from doctors to the paramedical professions, with the former group retaining a degree of overall control through membership of regulatory bodies such as the Council for Professions supplementary to Medicine.[23] The same approach to change continued and can be discerned in new legislation which will allow a limited degree of prescribing by nurses; the details are being negotiated with the medical profession.[24] This long-established pattern of change *between* occupations is, however, in the process of being superseded in importance by a pattern of change *within* professions. Although there has long been a degree of polarization whereby professionals transferred routine, 'unskilled', elements of their work to unqualified subordinate groups (such as nursing auxiliaries/assistants or physiotherapy aides), this new development is likely to be far more pervasive. This is best, though not uniquely, illustrated by the case of nursing, where three factors have come together to create radical change in the workforce in the form of semi-skilled 'health care assistants', able to undertake a good deal of nursing work but subject neither to the national requirements of licensure by the United Kingdom Central Council for Nursing, Midwifery and Health Visiting (UKCC), nor to any national arrangements for pay bargaining or review.

The first factor has been the drive by nurses themselves towards greater professionalization. There has long been a body of opinion within the profession advocating more extensive 'off-the-job' training, leading to a more advanced level of qualification. This movement found its first official recognition in government acceptance of the principles of the Briggs Report of 1972, and its belated implementation in the form of the Nurses, Midwives and Health Visitors Act 1979. This Act created the UKCC, which in turn developed Project 2000 to incorporate a good deal of Briggs' thinking, and is resulting in gradual but continuous shift towards degree-level nurse training. The concept of the 'new nursing', whilst more radical than the Briggs proposals is another manifestation of the same professionalizing drive.

The second factor contributing to radical change has been the presence of macro-level pressures *against* greater professionalization. One obvious such pressure is that of cost; a more highly trained workforce will not only be more expensive to produce but almost certainly more expensive to employ. Another such pressure is shortage of potential recruits; as we showed in Chapter 2, one result of contemporary demographic shifts is a significantly reduced proportion of population in the age groups from which student nurses (as well as entrants to the paramedical professions) have been recruited. Such pressure would be likely to be exacerbated by any raising of the minimum qualifications for entry to training.

The third factor has been an enabling one; the development since 1985 of the system of National Vocational Qualifications (NVQ) with the support of government, employers and the trades union movement. This system comprises arrangements for the national accreditation (at a range of levels) of vocational training undertaken for a wide range of pre-existing qualifications, as well as good quality training not otherwise recognized for qualifications. The system, which is a general one, and not confined to particular industries and occupations, permits individuals to build a recognized and coherent competency base for career progression by means of the principles of credit accumulation and transfer.[25]

It is the interaction between these three sets of factors that has permitted the establishment of the new occupation of health care assistant described above. This interaction has been summed up by one commentator as follows (Robinson 1992: 36):

An unholy alliance?

(. . .) Within nursing, the most recent debates have been about occupational closure; the professionalisers arguing for a high-status single portal, while the management have been concerned to open the entry gate to sustain the levels of nurses necessary to staff the service. However, on the organisation of the nursing workforce it would appear that the interests of the professionalisers and those of the employers may coincide. While the employers are concerned with the potential costs of a high-status elite profession, their worries are ameliorated by the creation of a flexible cheap peripheral workforce. This workforce consists currently of nurses qualified to both registered and enrolled nurse status and support workers. As the support workers' training acquires academic status and the worth of the qualified nurses' qualifications becomes eroded by time and comparison with Project 2000 Diplomates and degree nurses, it is difficult to see the distinction between the types of peripheral workers being sustained. This could force the cost of such workers downwards unless powerful union pressures oppose such a downward drift, and it is hard to see where such union pressure might come from.

**Box 3.3**  Occupational control in radiography

[Radiographers] are trained in schools normally located in hospitals and undertake practical experience in working radiology departments whilst receiving DHSS funded bursaries. The Radiographers Board of the Council for Professions Supplementary to Medicine (CPSM), recognises only one qualification for state registration, the Diploma of the College of Radiographers, and has the statutory authority to recognise training institutions and courses of training leading to the diploma. The College and Society of Radiographers are the product of a formal split between the educational and collective bargaining roles respectively of the former Society which occurred in 1978. The two bodies continue to share the same premises and it is not possible to be in membership of one without the other, a joint fee being payable.

The College of Radiographers specifies guidelines in terms of staff, facilities and maximum permitted student intakes to schools of radiography and it was by revision of these that the 1977 reduction in the number of radiography students was achieved. Hence the College/Society has effective unilateral control over the maximum number of students trained each year. Although in theory the Council and Board could recognise other qualifying bodies, the composition of the Board – a majority of radiographers are in practice College members – makes this unlikely. In addition, the highly technological requirements of radiographer training make a change to other institutions impractical.

*Source:* S. Harrison (1981) 'The politics of health manpower'. In Long, A.F. and Mercer, G. (eds) *Manpower Planning in the National Health Service*, 92–93. Gower, Farnborough.

In other words, the polarization of the nursing profession enhances its controllability by management. The same will turn out to be true of other health professions, too. Box 3.3 summarizes the rather obscure form of control which some professions (in this case, Radiography) have been able to exert over career prospects. NVQ will erode this control.

For those who remain within the élite, there are benefits, though experience so far suggests that the satisfactions of primary nursing will be unrealizable in the short term due to resistance by the medical profession.[26] This observation leads us directly into Chapter 4 and our consideration of the strategy of control which we have termed 'incorporation'.

# 4

# INCORPORATING THE
# PROFESSIONALS

We now turn to a more oblique approach to the management control of professionals than the 'head-on' approach which formed the subject matter of the preceding chapter. We refer to this approach as the 'incorporation' of professionals into management activity, and under this heading we shall be discussing resource management (RM) and its predecessors, doctors as managers and related clinical management structures, and the development of professionally-run audit and quality mechanisms. Each of these three closely related topics is the subject of a separate sub-section, in each of which (as in Chapter 3) we examine their theory, origins, content and effect. All these developments pre-date the White Paper *Working for Patients*, though, as we shall see in Chapter 5, the latter may well have a significantly enhancing effect.

Before beginning these substantive topics, however, we need to add a few words about the notion of 'incorporation' around which we have based this chapter. Until recent years, 'incorporation' has been a term used (mostly by academics) to describe the creation and maintenance of a particular set of relationships – close or even cosy relationships – between government and leading producer groups within a state (Schmitter 1974: 87):

> a system of interest representation in which the constituent units are organised into a limited number of singular, com-pulsory, non-competitive, hierarchically ordered categories, recognised or licensed (if not created by) the state and granted a deliberate representational monopoly . . . in exchange for

observing certain controls on their selection of leaders and articulating of demands and supports.

Hence, this general theoretical approach is known as *corporatism*. In it, both Parliament and political parties take side seats. The big deals are worked out between the state and the 'peak associations' (the favoured, élite, organized groups) and then 'sold' to the rank and file and the general public. Not all sectors of society are necessarily corporatized in this way, and in practice not every single one of Schmitter's criteria may be met even in those sectors where there is an élite interest group favoured by the state.

The relevance of all this for health policy is clear. The medical profession is surely just such a state-licensed élite – at least for the purposes of its national-level dealings with government. The state uses its legislative authority effectively to prohibit non-members of the profession from practising medicine, and the profession purports to control and discipline its members in return.[1]

In the last decade, however, scholars have begun to re-focus their observations about corporatism away from the national level implied by the above description, and towards the same kind of relationships at a more local level. In addition, corporatism has come to be seen less as a *theory* ('the state needs to come to an accommodation with powerful producer groups and is, in effect, compelled into the corporatist bargain') and more as a *description* of a set of relationships. Thus, corporatism could merely be a specific tactic employed by the state to keep powerful groups under control.[2]

It is this last sense in which we employ the notion of incorporation in this chapter, except that we have re-located it at the micro-level. Incorporation here refers to government/managerial tactics to control health professionals by encouraging some of them to become involved on managers' terms, in management processes which include a degree of control over their professional colleagues.[3]

## RESOURCE MANAGEMENT: PROFESSIONALS WITH BUDGETS

The notion that clinical professionals, especially doctors, should be internal budgetholders is more than twenty years old. Resource management (RM) is currently its most obvious manifestation. We

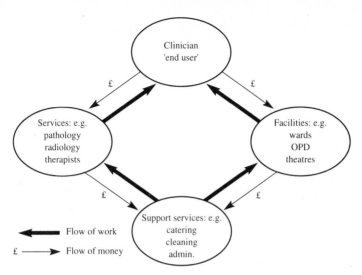

**Figure 4.1** Budgets for doctors: axioms. ('clinical budgets', 'management budgets', 'resource management')

shall briefly examine the history of this development in a moment, but let us first lay down the basic principles which underpin the idea; we shall see that there are important variations in systems, but that all are based on the axioms sketched out in Figure 4.1.[4]

The logic of Figure 4.1 can be summarized as follows:

- Clinical doctors (that is, those fully-qualified medical practitioners whose job is to provide therapy for patients), because they utilize their 'clinical freedom' (see Chapter 2) to accept patients, arrive at diagnoses, and decide upon treatment, are ultimately responsible for determining the use to which NHS resources are put. (For this reason they are sometimes termed 'clinical end users'.)
- Of course, such doctors do not work alone. They receive services, such as X-ray and pathology laboratory tests, which help to *diagnose* patients, *therapeutic* services such as physiotherapy, and *care* facilities, such as nursing, in locations such as wards, operating theatres and outpatient departments. Finally, there are *support services*, such as catering, cleaning, and maintenance, which are provided throughout the institution.
- 'Clinical end users' should therefore be holders of budgets,

related to their activity levels, against which internal charges should be levied in respect of the services received from other departments.

● The effect, therefore, is to create a set of explicit financial responsibilities and relationships within the institution.

The above logic, however, conceals a number of questions and assumptions which need to be explored. These can be divided into two groups: behavioural and technical. Let us first say something about the former.

As we have noted, RM assumes that it is meaningful to regard clinical doctors as 'end users', that is, they really do determine the distribution of resources between (types of) patient, as well as the number of patients treated. One objection to this is that doctors do not really make these decisions, but rather respond to the 'objective' needs of patients. This is both false and true: false because the patient's needs are not objective at all, but are subjectively recognized and acted upon by the doctor (as we saw in Chapter 2, some needs may be labelled as 'low priority' and not met) but true to the extent that there are very large numbers of patients in respect of whom there would be widespread medical (and lay) recognition that more-or-less immediate treatment is required.

A more indirect criticism of the basic RM axiom is that there are end users other than clinical doctors. Physiotherapists and chiropodists are often cited as cases in point. The latter are able to treat patients without any medical referral whatsoever. Most physiotherapy patients are referrals from doctors, but it is not customary in these cases for the doctor to specify what treatment should be given by the physiotherapist. There is, therefore, a question as to why the budget holding doctor should be financially responsible for the physiotherapist's treatment decisions; why should he or she 'sign a blank cheque'?

There is also a broader set of questions about the responsibility structure which is implied by RM. It seems clear that clinical end users are responsible for the *volume* of services and facilities that they use, whilst the heads of the departments that supply these are responsible for their (transfer) price. But these two factors are not unrelated to each other; since many of the service and facility departments (such as X-ray and hospital wards) have a high proportion of fixed and semi-fixed costs, changes in volume will affect unit costs. In particular, if budgetary considerations lead clinical doctors to reduce their usage of services and facilities, the result, other things being equal, will be a rise in the unit costs for the supplying department. It is, moreover, something of a moot point as to who is responsible for quality. Is it up to the end user to specify, or for the providing department to operate according to some professionally specified standards? (Many hospital laboratories, for instance, voluntarily subscribe to a nationally operated quality control scheme.) Or is the matter of quality simply not a feature of the system?

Another question is whether *individual* clinical doctors should be regarded as end users, or should be involved as groups or teams. As we shall see in the next section of this chapter, there are implications for the organization structure of the institution. Finally, why should doctors take part in such a system? One view might be that no incentive is, or should be, required; a management decision should be sufficient. But our discussion of professionalism in chapter 2 suggests that such an approach might be less than straightforward. A second view might be that extrinsic incentives might be offered; typically, this would take the form of *virement*, that is, of allowing budgetholders who underspend their budget to retain all or part of the savings for their departments or services. A third view is that RM offers *intrinsic* benefits, in the form of clinically interesting information, and a sense of control, to its participants.

If we now turn to the matter of technical assumptions, there are obvious questions about how both 'activity' and 'costs' are to be defined for the purposes of specific applications of RM.

How can clinical activity be defined? The simplest approach is to count 'cases', that is, in the context of hospital inpatients, dis-charges/deaths or, more recently, 'finished consultant episodes'. This is unlikely to be satisfactory for very long because it will aggregate together many different types of patient, often with very different workload and resource implications. In practice, there-fore, some notion of *casemix* has to be employed. Such casemix measures (of which the best known and most widely used are Diagnosis Related Groups – DRGs) aim to provide a classification system which groups together cases on the basis of their expected cost, or some proxy measure for it. Such 'iso-resource' groups thus serve as a measure of output from hospital beds. Figure 4.2 and Box 4.1 give an example of a group of DRGs.[5]

Some kind of definition of workload or activity is an obvious prerequisite of any attempt to make a budgetary allocation based

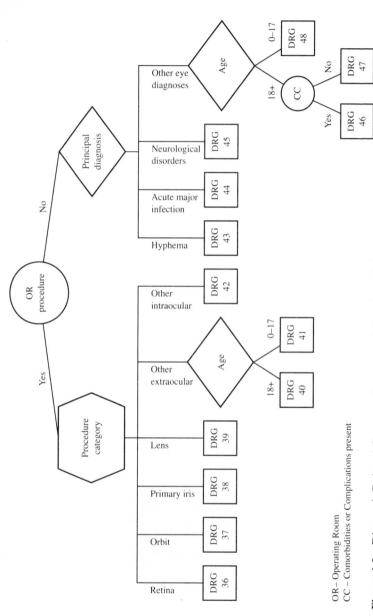

OR – Operating Room
CC – Comorbidities or Complications present

**Figure 4.2** Diagnosis Related Groups – diseases and disorders of the eye

*Source*: J. Coles (1986), 'The myths and realities of DRGs in the NHS', *Hospital and Health Services Review*, 82(1): 29. Reproduced by permission of the Institute of Health Services Management.

---

**Box 4.1**   A commentary on Figure 4.2

The DRG system begins its classification by concentrating on a broad group of diseases, often defined in respect of an organ system of the body. Figure 4.2 deals with diseases of the eye.

The classification process is in the form of an algorithm, beginning with whether or not the case is a surgical one. If surgery is involved (the left-hand branch of the figure) the site of the procedure is usually sufficient to determine the classification, though in one case age provides a further node in the algorithm.

The right-hand side of the algorithm is the non-surgical ('medical' in the narrow sense) area. In this case, the principal diagnosis (based on an international classification system) is the sole determinant of many DRGs. Again, age is involved in one branch of algorithm, as is the presence or absence of certain specified (not listed in the Figure) complications or additional diagnoses.

Remember that two patients classified to the same DRG will expect to consume the same amount of resources. There is a table of weightings (not shown) which shows the resource implications of DRGs relative to each other.

---

upon it. A further question then arises as to what elements of the costs of such activity are to be included in budgets, and hence be the subject of transfer charges within the hospital. At one end of the spectrum, the view could be adopted that only *direct* costs should be employed: these are defined as costs which are directly incurred by the budgetholder's decisions. (In the clinical context, these would be factors such as X-rays, laboratory tests, and drugs prescribed.) More broadly, budgets might also include *indirect* costs, such as staff salaries and wages, whilst at the opposite end of the spectrum the view might be taken to include an allocation of more remote indirect costs, such as heating, lighting and maintenance. Proponents of RM-like arrangements in the NHS have not always agreed about the most desirable approach. Put simply, the use only of direct costs is credible with budgetholders precisely because they are controllable; on the other hand, the inclusion of indirect costs can be defended on the grounds that might be expected to lead budgetholders to seek to influence them in the medium term.

Once decisions have been taken about the concepts of workload and cost to be employed in an RM system, information systems would have to be developed accordingly. The perceived accuracy of information inputs to the system would be expected to have an important bearing on its credibility to budgetholders and thereby upon their behavioural responses to both budgetary information and other information produced by the system. Although we have treated behavioural and technical assumptions which underpin RM separately over the last few pages, the two are, of course, intimately related. (We illustrated this in our discussion of performance indicators in Chapter 3.) Here are four further examples, related to RM:

- Defining activity in the medical sphere is technically quite complex. But doctors' own interests are likely to play a part in the adoption of definitions which are compatible with those interests; in turn, the definitions adopted, and their budgetary consequences, may impact upon the way in which cases are classified. This process is visible in the phenomenon known as 'DRG creep', observable in the Medicare system in the United States. Where there is uncertainty as to the primary diagnosis (as there often is) the tendency is to define the case as belonging to the Diagnostic Group yielding the highest reimbursement. Similarly, there may be an incentive to find and record complications or secondary diagnoses as a means of reclassifying the patient.
- It is possible to use information as a resource by which to induce behavioural change: we discussed the possibilities of both information as an *intrinsic* benefit to doctors and as a means to secure the *extrinsic* benefits of virement.
- There exist several possible technical approaches to defining the costs of activities. Each of these is likely to have a different impact on the behaviour of budgetholders. The inclusion of indirect costs in budgets is likely to lead to greater questioning of (for instance) staffing levels, especially if virement is offered as an incentive, than would occur if only direct costs were employed.
- There is a potentially two-way relationship between the accuracy of information and its use. It is a commonplace claim that particular pieces or sets of information are not used because they are inaccurate, but there is an equally plausible, though less

commonly heard, claim that the reverse is the case. In other words, there is an argument that the only way to improve inaccurate information is to begin to use it, so providing an incentive to improve accuracy.

It has been necessary to deal at some length with the theory and assumptions of RM. We can now briefly examine its history in the NHS. The development of RM can be seen in three phases: 'clinical budgets', 'management budgets', and after 1986, RM itself.

By the 1970s the established accounting systems within the NHS were such as to generate functional costs by institution or department. Thus it was possible to calculate the average cost per in-patient or per outpatient in a given hospital or by a given functional department (e.g. pathology, nursing, pharmacy, etc.). The production of such figures required little or no participation from clinicians, and the heads of functional departments frequently had little control over the expenditure charged to their budgets. For example, it would have been extremely unusual for a pharmacist to challenge a doctor's request for drugs on grounds of the expenditure thereby incurred.

From the early 1970s there were isolated and temporary experiments with alternative forms of budgeting, until in the early 1980s the Clinical Accountability, Service Planning and Evaluation Research Unit tried out *clinical budgets* in three health authorities. In these trials, teams of doctors and nurses were asked to accept responsibility for those expenditures which were directly related to patient care. They thus required far more active cooperation by clinicians than the orthodox functional costing system. As an incentive for taking on this extra responsibility the teams were allowed, within locally agreed rules, to employ savings in one area of their budget to finance expenditure in another.[6]

The impetus for *Management Budgets* (MB) came directly from the Griffiths Report, which recommended that health authorities should

. . . develop [MB] involving clinicians at unit level with the emphasis on management and not accountancy. The aim is to produce an unsophisticated system in which workload related budgets covering financial and manpower allocations and full overhead costs are closely related to workable service objectives, and against which performance and progress can be measured.

Thus, like clinical budgets, management budgets allocated resources to consultants and gave them specific responsibility for managing programmes of clinical care. MB however, made clinicians responsible for indirect as well as direct costs and did not necessarily allow underspending to be reallocated by the budget-holder.

In stark contrast to the approach favoured for other major managerial changes in the NHS, the then Department of Health and Social Security acknowledged that such a major development in budgeting as was heralded by MB needed to be demonstrated before it could be adopted across the country. The term 'demonstration' was used advisedly; a straight transfer to the public sector of a technique that had been an integral part of management in the private sector for over 40 years. Even before the publication of the Griffiths Report, four health authorities agreed to participate in demonstrations with a view to operating MB in a hospital setting during the financial year 1984–85. They were chosen partly because there were doctors in each of the areas who were favourably disposed towards MB, and while the basic philosophy of MB remained common across the four sites, the actual systems introduced into each differed slightly.

One of the firms of management consultants, in its review of developments in the MB demonstration sites, pointed to modest success, though most of their assertions lacked supporting evidence.[7] It was claimed that clinicians had accepted the principle of clinicians being budgetholders. It was also suggested that professionals had accepted that output could be measured. The management consultants argued that even crude output measures could produce reasonably accurate budgets and were useful as a first step in measuring performance.

The management consultants' review further claimed that uncomplicated information systems were able to produce MB data quickly and cheaply, which would facilitate the spread of MB and reduce the start-up costs; that accountants had learnt a new role and had moved away from the negative control aspects of accountancy to the positive provision of an information service to clinicians; and that, appropriate structures were evolving to enable MB to succeed. In particular, clearly-defined reporting structures were being established between clinicians and general managers.

Despite the limited gains in the deployment and management of resources, it is immediately clear from a review of the management consultancy reports on the first-generation MB initiative that attention had been concentrated almost exclusively on getting the technical systems in place and that insufficient attention had been given to winning the support of doctors and other professionals, on whom the success of the venture so crucially depended. Those involved in the exercise argued that what was required was better preparation of the ground so that hostilities and resistance were not aroused and genuine commitment was ensured. The means to achieve this would include discussions and seminars with all affected staff. Thus, the management consultants regarded this essentially as an implementation problem to be tackled by paying more attention to MB acceptance by all budgetholders including clinicians and general managers, and by involving other staff groups, like nurses, who had generally been excluded.

Despite the problems encountered in the first-generation MB demonstration sites, the DHSS decided to press on rapidly with a second-generation MB exercise. This was to be conducted in more than a dozen health districts, again in hospital settings, though in addition, proposals were invited for a demonstration project for community health services. In announcing its intentions the DHSS emphasized the need to give more attention to the behavioural aspects of introducing MB.

Subsequently, in November 1986, the Department produced a review of the combined experiences of the first and second generations.[8] The review conceded that some fundamental problems had not been overcome: a good technical foundation for MB had, apparently, been established, but there had been resistance and lack of enthusiasm on the part of medical staff. In an unusually candid passage for a departmental review in the public domain (DHSS, Health Notice (86)34, 1986, pp. 2, 5 and Appendix 1, pp. 1–2), the Department revealed that:

> Experience suggests that management arrangements which centrally involve doctors and nurses are a necessary precondition for effective management budgets . . . In the case of the four acute sites, the specialty and consultant costing and budgeting developments to date have so far not made a worthwhile contribution to the planning and costing of patient care . . . the net result is that many doctors, both at the demonstration sites and elsewhere, have still to be convinced that management budgeting is more than an accounting exercise

which simply increases overheads for no commensurate benefit
. . . in some districts where fundamental difficulties have been
encountered, or medical and nursing staff have been seriously
antagonised, there may be a case for suspending management
budgeting development for the time being.

To tackle these wider management dimensions, a third-generation
MB exercise was announced in November 1986. It involved six hospital service sites and several community health service sites. The
term 'resource management' was employed in preference to MB to
reflect the renewed emphasis on management rather than budgeting: this approach was pointedly described as a wider approach
which would emphasize 'medical and nursing ownership of the
system'. No attempt was made precisely to distinguish it from MB.

Given the acknowledgement that doctors had often not found the
earlier MB experiments credible, it was not surprising that, in
launching RM, great care was taken to secure the agreement of representatives of the medical profession. This agreement involved a
commitment to evaluate the pilot sites prior to any further extension of the RM initiative; the evaluation was published in late 1991,
though a decision had long before been announced to extend RM as
part of the subsequent *Working for Patients* reforms which we discuss in Chapter 5.

What, then, has been the impact of RM upon relationships between managers and health professionals? In general, the RM pilot
site evaluation shows evidence of managerial benefits such as improvements in resource allocation and increases in efficiency. It is
clear, though, that RM has by no means provided a pervasive means
of control of doctors. One reason for this is that the dissemination of
RM has been relatively slow; even after the long history which was
summarized above, there is still no hospital the whole of whose
clinical activity is covered by RM. Another reason for the limited
impact of RM is the paradox that it cannot be implemented without
the cooperation (or more) of doctors themselves. One way of se-
curing this cooperation has been to allow doctors the major say in
the content of the information system which supports RM. But the
inevitable outcome is information which is of primary interest to
clinicians rather than managers, and the pilot site evaluation suggests that by 1991, and in marked contrast to the situation in 1986
(see above) or even 1988, doctors tended to have positive views of
RM.[9]

Thus, it is possible that the restricted impact of RM may be a short-term phenomenon; once systems are in place, they may increasingly affect professionals' behaviour without the need for managerial intervention. Let us give two examples. The first example concerns 'creeping developments'. This phrase refers to a situation where medical developments, such as a surgeon's decision to use a particular kind of artificial hip joint, or to treat more of a particular kind of patient, lead to unplanned expenditure increases which managers only find out about after the event. In principle, RM might be expected both to provide managers with early evidence of such 'creep' and also to signal to doctors that such evidence would be available and therefore that they should discuss with managers the expenditure consequences of changes in medical practice in advance. Although there is some evidence of success in this respect from *management budgeting* sites, the Brunel evaluation of the *RM* pilot sites noted that cost awareness still relied upon initiatives from general management that pre-dated the RM experiment, rather than being generated by the service providers themselves. As we shall see in Chapter 5, later NHS changes may significantly enhance the behavioural impact of RM.

The second example concerns the possibility that RM may provide a common, agreed factual base upon which doctors and managers can argue about what decisions should be taken. There is considerable evidence from the RM pilot sites that the system is capable of functioning in this way. But, of course, this does not necessarily create the situation in which the professionals become self-managing. Box 4.2 illustrates the point; the information is agreed, but views about what action should be taken vary wildly.

The story may be different for nurses, however. Although the early RM tended to marginalize nursing management, subsequent spread of RM has been accompanied by much greater involvement. RM has now become very much associated with the nurse staffing control measures which we discussed in the preceding chapter, and is therefore much more of a traditional managerial control device over clinical nurses than over clinical doctors.

Increasingly, RM has become difficult to separate from other organizational changes within hospitals, and in particular from the strong trend towards the creation of new, clinically defined, structures of management. These are the topic of our next section.

**Box 4.2**    Consultants meeting in a directorate – October 1989

Present: clinical direction, four other consultants, senior registrar, business manager, researcher.

*Item – varicose veins*
The clinical director produced information regarding the monthly additions to the waiting lists for both inpatients and day patients. He and a second consultant agreed to reduce the day case waiting list by treating two or three extra cases each month. The clinical director then proposed reducing the inpatient list by creating a special waiting list of patients who were prepared to be admitted at short notice if there was a gap in theatre lists. The third consultant argued that this would not help. You could not solve problems by *ad hoc* measures, filling a vacant slot. It was necessary to draw up plans to take three extra inpatient admissions each month. The second consultant said that he could not participate in this. The third and fourth consultants felt that they could, although the latter wondered if the financial position meant that they could reduce varicose vein cases? The clinical director argued that hopefully the financial crisis (which he was coming to later) was a short-term problem, whereas reducing the waiting list was a matter of principle. The second consultant wondered if a registrars' varicose vein list could be treated on Monday mornings when there was a free theatre session? The clinical director agreed to investigate and check if an anaesthetist was available. The fifth consultant warned that the theatre was used for teaching purposes at this time and was not, in fact, available. The clinical director would investigate. The third consultant stressed that reducing the waiting list was a priority. The fifth consultant proposed adopting 'a blitz strategy' to get the waiting list down to an acceptable level. He was supported by the third consultant who also suggested that some of the figures relating to varicose vein operations were wrong. The clinical director asked the business manager to check the figures. The fourth consultant reminded the meeting that 'a blitz' on the waiting list would require additional funds. The clinical director agreed to investigate the possibility of additional finance from the current central government initiative being available.

*Source:* T. Packwood *et al.* (1992) *Hospitals in Transition*, 95. Open University Press, Buckingham.

## CLINICAL MANAGEMENT STRUCTURES

Doctors have in some sense been involved in management since the inception of the NHS in 1948. Some, especially in psychiatric hospitals, were career 'medical superintendents', combining clinical work with a permanent management position. Until the re-organization of 1974, Medical Officers of Health were effectively general managers of the various health service activities of local government authorities. In addition, considerable attention was given, from the late 1960s onwards, to how rank-and-file clinical doctors could be involved in the management process without themselves becoming managers. These, and subsequent developments can be seen as falling into three categories.[10]

First, there is the *career manager*; as noted above, the medical superintendent and Medical Officer of Health fell into this category, and so did those medically qualified persons appointed to general manager posts following the Griffiths Report of 1983. As Table 3.4 showed, some 15 per cent of the first round of general manager appointments went to doctors, though these were largely concentrated at the Unit (operational) level of organization, where almost one third of such posts were medically occupied, usually on a part-time basis alongside continuing clinical work. It appears that many of these have now returned to whole-time clinical work.[11]

A second category is the *accidental part-time manager*; such doctors are those who, by virtue of seniority or of roles as directors of clinical programmes, achieve a degree of authority amongst their colleagues. It can be argued that these are at the same time the most influential but underestimated players in the medical management system. But precisely because their role is contingent and 'accidental', it has not been the subject of management policy.

The third category is the *management-prone* specialist, that is a senior consultant working in an organizational context where management of non-medical staff is important, and where a high degree of integration with other parts of the organization is required. Such conditions have long applied, for instance, in hospital pathology and radiology departments. However, the important development which forms the topic of this section is, in effect, the deliberate manipulation of organization structures so that the above requirements apply more widely than just to the kinds of department cited. This new development may be termed the 'clinical directorate'.

In order to understand the potential significance of these new

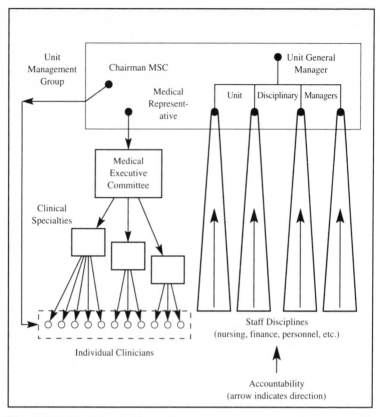

**Figure 4.3**   The traditional hospital organization structure (MSC = Medical Staff Committee)

*Source:* T. Packwood *et al.* (1992) 'Process and structure: resource management and the development of sub-unit organisational structure', *Health Services Management Research*, 5(1).

forms of hospital management structures, we begin by outlining the traditional, functional-professional structures which they replace. A typical example of the traditional arrangement is shown at Figure 4.3.

It can readily be seen that the key features of this arrangement are twofold. First, there is a heavy reliance on *profession* as an organizing principle. Doctors are organized through the committee structure at the left-hand side of Figure 4.3, whilst the other health professions (and some management specialties too) are organized in a set of discrete hierarchies shown at the right.[12] Second, it will be seen that, so far as doctors are concerned, accountability flows in the opposite director from the usual hierarchy, with the Medical Executive Committee responsible to the rank and file.

A typical view of the effects of this traditional structure is as follows (Packwood *et al.* 1992: 68–70).

> The structure relied upon communication via hierarchical chains of management or transmission by the medical representatives. Neither could easily combine the aggregate and strategic approach required for unit-level resource management, with the detailed and operational approach required in providing services to individual patients. For one thing, because it was based upon functional disciplines, management was necessarily focussed on staff inputs, admittedly vital and expensive, into the provision of patient treatment and care. This focus fragmented the approach to treatment, which usually required the contribution of a number of disciplines, and made treatment processes all the harder to manage. It also made it harder to think about the work in terms of processes and outputs for patients . . . Management based upon staff disciplines tended, inevitably, to be somewhat introverted. It was also difficult in that, although hierarchical staff accountability did finally come together at unit level in the role of the general manager, representative accountability in the medical discipline moved in the opposite direction, fragmenting out to the individual clinicians who occupied a collegial or peer relationship between themselves based upon personal power rather than managerial authority.
>
> In these circumstances it might prove tempting, and in some cases more productive, for individuals at the respective extremes to bypass the intermediate structure and relate directly; for unit general managers to undertake their own service negotiations with individual consultants, and for the latter to engage in service politics in pressing their own needs with senior unit managers.

In short, the structure worked against the integration of services for patients, and failed to provide much managerial control over doctors. By contrast the clinically-based hospital management structures which we are about to examine sought to incorporate doctors into the management process.

As with some of the ideas which we shall be examining in Chapter 5, these new forms of hospital management structure seem to originate in the United States, and indeed are sometimes referred to as the 'Johns Hopkins model' after the Baltimore teaching hospital where such forms were pioneered in the mid 1970s. The essence of the Johns Hopkins model is the constitution of a number of 'clinical units' within the hospital, defined in terms of specialty, and each managed by a medically qualified chief in a small management team of him or herself, a nurse director, and an administrator.[13] This management team has a budget, being accountable for direct costs, and (in principle at least) being able to choose between the purchase of centrally-provided catering, cleaning and maintenance services and their purchase from outside the hospital. In this model, the hospital becomes a kind of holding company for a series of specialty hospitals. Those involved at Johns Hopkins explicitly relate the model to what they regard as standard industrial practice, and are explicit in saying that it was devised in order to reduce hospitals costs (in the face of pressure from third party payers) by reducing lengths of inpatient stay in favour of more outpatient diagnosis and treatment.

The earliest importation of these ideas to the NHS seems to have been the experiment begun in 1984 at Guy's Hospital in the face of major financial problems. As two of the leading proponents of the scheme explained (Smith and Chantler 1987: 14), the necessity was seen as:

> to reconcile clinical freedom with management authority and accountability . . . the consultants agreed to accept a system that sought to equate power with responsibility. In return for the freedom to manage their own affairs, they had to accept responsibility for the financial consequences.

In the NHS context, the Johns Hopkins model, as implemented at Guy's and elsewhere, is termed the 'clinical directorate model', and is typified in Figure 4.4. In this model, the clinical director (usually, but not invariably, a member of consultant medical staff who continues to undertake part-time clinical work) is responsible to the hospital general manager, and is a budgetholder for the directorate. The directorate incorporates other health professionals working in the functional area which defines it. Clinical directors are normally assisted by one or more dedicated full-time managers, often from a nursing background. The position of the clinical director in such a

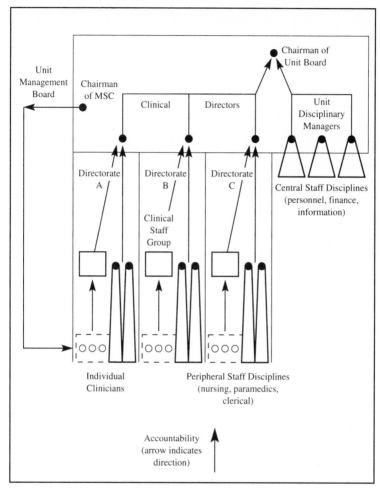

**Figure 4.4**  Clinical directorates in the NHS: a typical structure

*Source:* T. Packwood *et al.* (1992) 'Process and structure: resource management and the development of sub-unit organisational structure', *Health Services Management Research*, 5(1).

structure has been neatly summed up as follows (Packwood *et al.* 1992: 71–72):

> In addition to being able to 'hunt with the service providers', the clinical director must also 'run with the unit managers' and

along with fellow directors and senior unit disciplinary managers, contribute to determining unit plans and priorities as a member of the unit management board. This means acting as a corporate manager rather than as a representative of a particular directorate . . .

It is deemed essential that clinical directors are acceptable to both the consultant staff and to the management board and/or its chairman. This reflects the reality that they will be obliged to work in two modes: the political mode in leading their medical colleagues in the peer group, and the bureaucratic mode in managing the non-medical staff and contributing to unit management.

Although there seems to be little systematic evidence available, it seems clear that the clinical directorate model, or some variant of it, has become the preferred mode of organization of acute hospital units in the NHS. The variants may, in fact, be crucial transitional stages towards the full clinical directorate model illustrated in Figure 4.4. The flavour of the main form of variant is given in Figure 4.5. This takes the form of a two-dimensional matrix organizational structure for the hospital. It employs clinical specialties (or groups of them) as one dimension, and (non-medical) professional disciplines as the other. This arrangement provides a forum for the integration of services as they affect the patient. It is fairly clear, however, that they do not offer the same degree of authority to heads of groupings as the full Johns Hopkins model provides to clinical directors; their potential for managerial control over professionals is therefore much less. Of course, if it transpires that this variant is, in fact, a transitional stage towards the full model, then this will only be a temporary phenomenon.

The clinical directorate model is too new to the UK for any systematic research evidence about its impact to have become available. Indeed, it is still difficult to be sure about the precise extent of its diffusion, though this is certainly extensive in acute hospitals, but much less so in fields such as community services and mental illness.[14] Certainly the model appears to be popular with both clinicians and managers, though perhaps for different reasons. From the medical viewpoint

> Doctors must play a bigger part in managing the health service, to protect their clinical freedom.
>
> (Smith *et al.* 1989: 311)

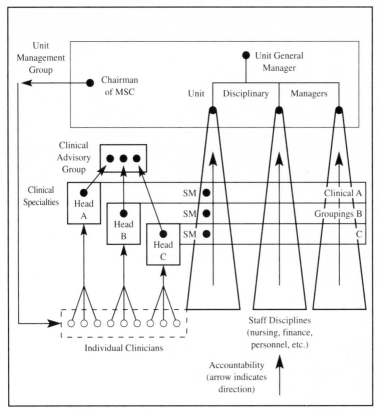

**Figure 4.5** Clinical groupings: matrix structures as a transitional stage (SM = Service Manager)

*Source:* T. Packwood *et al.* (1992) 'Process and structure: resource management and the development of sub-unit organisational structure', *Health Services Management Research*, 5(1).

> Doctors must run the NHS. Non-medical managers simply will not understand what health care is necessary.
>
> (Parkhouse *et al.* 1988: 25)

From the management viewpoint, however, the *raison d'être* of such models of organization includes greater managerial control over both doctors and other health professionals.[15] The vehicle for this control is the incorporation of professionals themselves into managerial roles, subject to managerial parameters, such as budgets; it begins to replace both the collegial assumptions which have underpinned the past organization of hospital medicine, and the closed managerial promotion system which has characterized the other health professions. The changes thus build on the belief, mentioned above, that if professionals do not become involved in management, it will be 'done to them', as indeed may well be the case. One way of seeing this is as a change in 'organizational culture' along the lines proposed in a currently best-selling management textbook:

> Psychologists study the need for self-determination in a field called 'illusion of control'. Stated simply, its findings indicate that if people think they have even modest personal control over their destinies, they will persist at tasks. They will do better at them. They will become more committed to them. . . . The fact . . . that we *think* we have a *bit* more discretion leads to *much* greater commitment.
>
> (Peters and Waterman 1982: 80–81, original emphasis)

In the language of political science/sociology, this equates to Lukes' 'third dimension' of power (Lukes 1974: 24):

> . . . is it not the supreme and most insidious exercise of power to prevent people, to whatever degree, from having grievances by shaping their perceptions, cognitions and preferences in such a way that they accept their role in the existing order of things, either because they can see or imagine no alternative to it, or because they see it as natural and unchangeable, or because they value it as divinely ordained and beneficial?

It is easy to see how clinical directorates are a logical sequel to RM, and we shall see in Chapter 5 how they may well be a crucial facilitating element in the 'purchaser/provider split' in health care. Before that, however, we have to conclude this chapter by dealing with another aspect of incorporation: the development of various approaches to 'quality' assessment and assurance in the NHS.

## QUALITY ASSESSMENT AND ASSURANCE IN THE HEALTH PROFESSIONS

Matters of quality are not wholly new to the NHS. Institutions such as the Health Advisory Service date back to the long stay hospital scandals of the 1960s.[16] However, it was during the late 1980s and early 1990s that 'quality' became an extraordinarily widely used term within NHS and other public service contexts. The Health Service experienced a veritable epidemic of Total Quality Management schemes, quality circles, Directors of Quality Assurance, quality standards (including all the fuss around BS5750), quality charters and the like.[17] A commonplace professional reaction to this quality 'hype' was the faintly defensive observation that health care professionals have always been strongly focussed on the quality of their work, and that it was misleading to imply that such concerns were in any way new.

What is actually going on here, we suggest, is a struggle for control, very much including control of the meaning of the terms and labels used to describe and define the services the NHS provides. If incorporation is a strategy for involving professional producer groups in sharing management responsibilities with the state then the most profound level of such a strategy is the creation of shared *meanings*. Thus arguments over definitions and purposes are anything but 'academic'. On the contrary the new prominence (and new meanings) given to 'quality' can be regarded as part of a highly political process. It is therefore pertinent to enquire *who* is pressing for increased attention to quality, and *how* that quality is defined.

Of course, we do *not* mean that all the activity around 'quality' is no more than a cynical battle for 'turf'. Clearly much of the effort going into quality improvement of one kind or another is relatively altruistic, genuinely directed at improving citizens' experiences of their National Health Service. Yet however well-meaning individual 'improvers' may be they are nonetheless obliged to adjust their efforts so that they conform to the prevailing contours of power, authority and autonomy within their respective health care organizations. When in 1989 the Association of Community Health Councils for England and Wales asked to be formally represented in the process of medical audit the Department of Health (DoH) indicated that this would not be appropriate because medical audit was a professional exercise. Medical quality, in other words, was not Community Health Council (CHC) turf, it was doctors' turf. The renewed interest in quality over the last few years has thrown up numerous examples of similar territorial sensitivity. After all, as we pointed out in Chapter 1, the first, 'functional' notion of professionalism sees the determination of standards as a quintessentially intra-professional task, not one to be much shared with either the client/patient or, indeed, with management.

It may be worth adding an acknowledgement here that our following exploration of quality is of a particularly limited and focussed kind. We will *not* be attempting to establish which quality technique is the 'best', which measurement techniques are reliable and valid or which local schemes have commanded the highest commitment from NHS staff. Nor will we be seeking answers to any number of other important evaluatory questions. Our more modest ambition is to understand the ways in which the current quest for 'quality' seems likely to impinge on professional autonomy, professional/management relationships and the more general organization of work in the NHS of the near future.

To begin with, then, we will analyse the contested issue of definitions, titles and meanings. This can be fairly closely related to lines of occupational demarcation. Once we have cleared a little semantic space we will then proceed to compare and contrast three different approaches to health service quality: medical audit, nursing quality initiatives and Total Quality Management schemes (TQM).

The term 'quality' has come to be used in a bewilderingly promiscuous way. The literature includes references to 'quality' inputs (e.g. fully-trained nurses; high-tech medical equipment), 'quality' processes (e.g. following the appropriate clinical protocol), 'quality' outputs (e.g. low wound infection rates) and 'quality' outcomes (e.g. low infant mortality rates, high quality-weighted five-year surgical survival rates). Figure 4.6 indicates the relationships between some of the main performance terms.

Quality improvements are said to include such diverse activities as introducing floral duvets in the geriatric ward, liberalizing visiting hours, offering more choice on hospital menus, carrying out patient satisfaction surveys, participating in the National Confidential Enquiry into Perioperative Deaths, holding medical audit meetings, persuading consultants to liaise more closely with local GPs, writing certain patient's 'rights' into the contracts by which health authorities purchase services from providers and, of course, the *Patients' Charter*.[18]

There are a variety of ways of making sense of this seemingly infinite variety. We particularly notice that 'quality' as an issue within the NHS was quickly divided up along 'tribal' lines. Thus in the mid-1980s many health authorities appointed 'Directors of Quality Assurance' or the like, most of them with a nursing background. These individuals were subsequently given responsibility

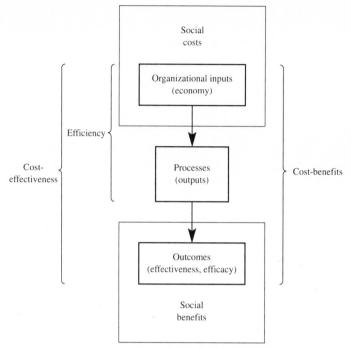

**Figure 4.6**   Performance terms in medical care organizations

*Source:* S. Harrison (1992) 'Management and doctors'. In Bhugra, D. and Burns, A. (eds) *Management Training for Psychiatrists*. Gaskell, London.

for 'total quality' schemes and various other initiatives, but very seldom for the quality of *medical* activities. This latter area was effectively hived off as the exclusive preserve of doctors themselves. The white paper largely maintained this distinction, the Working Paper on audit stating that:

> The Government's approach is based firmly on the principle that the quality of medical work can only be reviewed by a doctor's peers.

This was not a principle applied by the Government to any other type of health care work. It led to semantic curiosities, such as the Government's funding of 17 pilot 'Total Quality Management' schemes whose concerns were actually total quality *minus* medical quality, a hollow-centred totality.

Yet even within the NHS TQM schemes 'quality' was still over-whelmingly defined by the service *providers* themselves, be they nurses, physiotherapists, receptionists, medical records clerks or whatever. At the time of writing it remains rare for final users – patients, potential patients and their relatives – to have much say in the definition of quality. This would seem strange to some quality experts from the private sector, where quality is not infrequently defined as 'fitness for purpose'. For the 'purpose' referred to in this phrase is meant to be that of the consumer, not the provider's. Private sector firms are increasingly likely to expend some consider-able effort in order to find out exactly what the consumer's purposes are.

Thus it would not be too much of an exaggeration to say that, in terms of the dominant 'players' actually involved, there are actually at least three species of 'quality' abroad in the NHS of the early 1990s. First, there is *medical quality*, the definition of which remains a professional and often highly technical exercise conducted exclus-ively by doctors. Second, there is what we might term *service quality*, which comprises the many aspects of providing health care services which remain once 'doctors' business' has been artificially extracted. In practice discussions of service quality tend to be dominated by the providers themselves, and especially by nurses and managers. (To be fair it should be pointed out that the prime 'customers' for many health service providers are other health service providers, e.g. when a laundry provides a ward with fresh linen or a pathology laboratory carries out tests for a consultant.) Finally there is the user's *experienced quality*. This is the type of quality we currently know least about. Of course, patient satisfac-tion surveys are beginning to dispel the murk, but even these may not capture all the dimensions of the experience which the patient thinks important, especially if the questionnaires are composed by managers rather than users themselves.

In the remainder of this section we look at three specific manifes-tations of the search for quality – medical audit, nursing quality and TQM schemes. These have been chosen mainly because they are currently the labels under which probably the greatest activity and discussion is taking place. We will relate each of these to the foregoing discussion of definitions and labels.

We begin with *medical audit*. A *prima facie* case for some form of this has long existed in the knowledge that there are large, un-explained, variations in practice between individual clinicians. This case has long been recognized in some sections of the medical

---

**Box 4.3**   The problems of clinical consensus

The clinician unlike the basic scientist has to act even when knowledge is insufficient for a fuller informed decision. A 'consensus' view under these circumstances can be achieved in only three ways: by compromise, by selection of an expert panel whose views conform, or by use of language that obscures differences.

When there are genuine differences of opinion in a review panel, compromise is the only way in which apparent unanimity can be obtained. The objection to describing the result as a consensus is that the term carries an authority that 'compromise guidelines' would not. Bias in selection of a review panel is unlikely to be intentional, but nevertheless carries an important risk. Distinction in medical science reflects prevailing values and prejudices; the minority questioning voice may well not be selected, although it may belong to tomorrow's majority.

. . . The rather heavy-handed style of clinical guideline documents is not entirely the fault of their semi-official status. Carefully selected words are an excellent way to obscure meaning – or the lack of it. The final report may misrepresent the keen debate that preceded it.

Editorial, *The Lancet* (1992), 339, 1197–8.

---

profession, and has led to a number of audit initiatives quite unconnected with management. Some such initiatives have been local; thus, a group of Edinburgh surgeons seem both to have constructed an impressive information and audit system concerning their own practice, and to have acted upon its implications. Similar behaviour changes resulting from audit have been reported in GPs' treatment of children.[19]

Other initiatives have been national in character, though still within the medical profession. One example has been the production of clinical guidelines, often by some sort of consensus process, though the effect of such guidelines on clinical practice is far from clear; as the *British Medical Journal* (1992: 305, 785) noted:

Writing them is easier than making them work.

---

**Box 4.4**    The Confidential Enquiry into Perioperative Deaths

This Enquiry was a joint venture between the Royal College of Surgeons and the Association of Anaesthetists. The Enquiry investigated all deaths within 30 days of surgery in three English regions in 1986. Reports on deaths were prepared by the doctors involved and these reports were independently assessed by relevant experts. An overall death rate of 0.7 per cent in over 500 000 operations was found. Death was attributed to avoidable surgical and anaesthetic factors in around 20 per cent of patients. A number of causes of concern were identified in the Enquiry report. These included: inadequate supervision of junior doctors by consultants; surgeons performing operations outside their main area of expertise; and surgeons and anaesthetists not holding regular audits of their operation results. On the basis of these findings, a series of recommendations were formulated with the aim of improving the quality of care. CEPOD was extended to England as a whole in 1988 with financial support from the DHSS.

*Source:* C. Ham and D.J. Hunter (1988) *Managing Clinical Activity in the NHS.* King's Fund Institute, London.

---

Perhaps this is not surprising; Box 4.3 graphically illustrates some of the weaknesses implicit in the whole notion of clinical consensus.[20] Another example of a national audit initiative from within the medical profession was the Confidential Enquiry into Perioperative Deaths, outlined in Box 4.4. This pilot arrangement was followed up by National CEPOD in 1989, though the evaluation method was modified to one based on comparing cases of death with a matched random sample of patients who survived similar surgery.[21]

All these initiatives were entirely voluntary – there was no question of health authorities, managers or anyone else *requiring* doctors to indulge in audit. *Working for Patients* changed this at a stroke. Henceforth, according to the Department of Health, Welsh Office, Scottish Home and Health Department and Northern Ireland Office, *Working for Patients* (1989: 40):

> Every consultant should participate in a form of medical audit
> agreed between management and the profession locally.

Similarly, GPs were expected to practise audit. In their case something similar had been advocated for several years by their forward-looking Royal College.

At first sight this might appear to constitute a major strengthening of external control of the medical profession. After all, a practice (medical audit) which had formerly been an occasional and voluntary activity by a minority of doctors was overnight transformed into virtually a mandatory practice by all doctors. In reality, however, the change was much less dramatic. In the medical audit Working Paper which followed *Working for Patients*, the Government conceded the 'principle that the quality of medical work can only be reviewed by a doctor's peers'. And during the months following the publication of *Working for Patients*, the profession worked hard to recapture the initiative. Several royal colleges rushed into print with audit guidelines.[22] Taken together these could be said to have created a *medical* model of medical audit, a version of audit which kept it as a non-threatening activity carried out only by doctors and rigorously protected from the public gaze.

This medical model comprised at least six main features:

(a) Only doctors should conduct audit.
(b) Its main purpose should be educational and developmental, *not* regulatory or judgemental.
(c) Participation should be voluntary and non-attendance should not be penalized.
(d) Standards should be set locally – by participating doctors.
(e) Absolute confidentiality should prevail.
(f) Where doctors regularly fell short of locally-determined standards this should be dealt with by medical peers, not as a management problem.

This version of audit is clearly not the only possible one. In the USA *external, regulatory* audit is conducted on a very large scale as a legal requirement of the Medicare programme. Internal medical audit also exists, but has been deemed insufficient by itself for the purposes of public accountability. External Professional Review Organisations (PROs) therefore hire doctors to act as physician reviewers, and the results of systematic reviews of participating institutions are available in the public domain. In the NHS there is, in effect, no external review.

Whilst the DoH and local management did not simply swallow the medical model wholesale neither did they appear to put up a very spirited resistance to the medical profession's bid to reassert control. It has to be remembered that 1989–90 was a period during which the Department and the organs of the medical profession were in open conflict over many of the elements of *Working for Patients*. Undoubtedly there was a sense in which both sides were relieved to find, in medical audit, a less controversial issue on which the usual processes of mutual adjustment and compromise could operate. As one medical negotiator said to us of the White Paper, 'We were grappling to find something we could see as good in it.'

Thus, of the six features of the medical model listed above, (a), (b) and (d) seemed to be conceded by the Department without much in the way of alternative suggestions. Voluntariness, however, was a sensitive issue. Significantly none of the official documents actually used the words 'mandatory' or 'compulsory'. In negotiation over the draft circulars the BMA managed to persuade the DoH that no new disciplinary procedure was required to deal with non-attenders. In other words the Government proceeded on the assumption that all doctors would heed the call but agreed not to use the inflammatory language of compulsion or to introduce any specific penalties for those who resisted.

On the issue of confidentiality the medical profession was able to point to the strict protection that had surrounded previous exercises and to argue that anything less than total anonymity would open doctors to malpractice litigation and therefore lead to widespread non-participation. (Whether there *should* be more malpractice litigation was a point seldom addressed.) Most health authorities quickly adopted formal codes of confidentiality, some of which openly adjured health authorities to take every possible step to deny information to patients who sought it. Those who attempted a more liberal approach soon encountered resistance. In one teaching district the chair of the medical audit group tried to introduce a respected member of the local Community Health Council (CHC) on to the committee. The surgeons immediately withdrew on the grounds that confidentiality was at risk.

The one point of 'leakage' in a process otherwise hermetically sealed against the non-medical world was the passing of 'aggregate data' from the District Medical Audit Group to local management.

By the beginning of 1992 this seemed to have been accepted – in principle – by the BMA and other medical bodies. However, not much actual transfer had yet taken place, and even acceptance in principle depended on total anonymity.

The final claim of the 'medical model' was that persistent medical underperformance was a medical, not a management problem. The key issue, therefore, concerns behavioural change. It is one thing to show that a group of clinicians committed to audit can change their practice, but quite another to show that such change can be obtained amongst the less committed.[23] At present, few managers seem inclined to make behavioural change an issue of principle, but rather await a suitable test case and meanwhile to avoid an unnecessary policy clash with the BMA. At the same time the BMA line was that the General Medical Council was reconsidering procedures for disciplining incompetence, that it was early days and that the rest of the NHS should await the outcome of these august (and long drawn-out) deliberations.

Whilst the policy stances of the Department, the BMA and the royal colleges are obviously important it is also necessary to ask what was going on at the grass roots. Here it is difficult to generalize, since at the time of writing audit was still only getting underway in many provider units. In most districts audit was treated as exclusively a professional development or educational activity. In some the audit sessions seemed to be being used mainly as an additional opportunity for consultants to instruct junior doctors. In one or two teaching hospitals earmarked audit money was in effect being regarded as a new way of funding little research projects. In many places the funds were being eagerly seized in order to appoint 'audit coordinators' who would gather data and help present it back to doctors. In none that we are aware of was the output of aggregate data to management or into the contracting process treated as a prime aim of the exercise. Indeed, the predominance of 'home-grown' local approaches to data collection meant that inter-unit or inter-district comparability was going to be difficult if not impossible. On the other hand a number of early successes were claimed – typically references to consultant colleagues who had changed their clinical practice after considering audit data. Those who refused to participate, or to heed the polite nudging of colleagues presented a much more difficult issue. As one audit group chair put it: 'Retraining and re-education are not yet part of the British version of the medical career.'

In sum, it may be said that in the short term, the medical profession has so far been largely successful in its attempt to shape and control medical audit in its own interests. In this sense 'medical quality' remains firmly the business of the doctor, not the patient (and not even the nurse, paramedic or manager). In the medium term, however, there is still potential for developing the audit process in such a way that it would begin to serve a somewhat wider range of interests. At least two crucial (and interrelated) points are likely to arise.

First, there is the probable desire of purchasing authorities for quality data in a form that permits them to compare one provider with another. The issue to be faced is inter-provider comparability. Even anonymous data can still be made comparable with (equally anonymous) data from other providers, thus enabling purchasers to 'rate' provider *units*, one against another. The logic of the provider market would appear to point to the desirability of exactly this type of comparison taking place. Yet, at the time of writing we are not aware of any such attempt other than a vague intention to compare hospital re-admission rates at some unspecified future time.[24] If and when purchasers are able to conduct quality comparisons in this way then a potentially important lever of influence will have been added to managers' armoury.

Second, there is the question of incentives or sanctions for provider quality performance which falls below the levels specified in the relevant contract or service agreement. Anecdotally we are aware that this second problem is already being faced in some districts, but it is not yet clear whether such problems will be acted on or brushed under the carpet. This may be partly influenced by degree of competition existing in the particular service in the particular locality. Where there is a realistic alternative provider the purchaser's hand will, *ceteris paribus*, be that much stronger.

Finally it would be wrong entirely to discount some 'internal', intra-professional tightening-up of medical audit. Some specialties and some districts have audit chairs who are vigorous and determined in their pursuit of high professional standards of self-appraisal. There are also those in the royal colleges who have fully accepted the strength of the case for audit. We have met some who insist, for example, on identifying outcome indicators and on comparing local performance with larger bodies of data. Perhaps even more important, some audit committees have created monitoring systems which show whether colleagues' clinical practices are actually changing as a result of audit or not. This may still be within the medical model, but at least is likely to be *effective* audit rather than just a talking shop.

We now move on to discuss nursing audit. The year 1989 did not mark such a sharp watershed for the audit of the quality of nursing as it did for medical audit. During the 1970s a range of ready-made systems had begun to travel eastwards across the Atlantic (e.g. Phaneuf Nursing Audit, Qualpacs and Monitor, an Anglicized version of the American Rush Medicus method) and (a later arrival) Excelcare. From the mid-1980s onwards a substantial number of DHAs set up Directorships of Quality Assurance (or posts with similar titles) and usually filled them with nurses.[25] By the beginning of 1989 many NHS hospitals already had in place systems for measuring various aspects of nursing work.

Whilst most of these systems are, like medical audit, mono-professional, there are important respects in which their application and development has been very different from that of medical audit. In particular:

- There has been less concentration (though still some) on issues of membership of committees, rules of confidentiality, etc. and more on the exact, step-by-step procedures to be followed in carrying out the audit.
- The detailed products of nursing audit have frequently been available to management. This is related to the next point.
- Nursing audit has been carried out in a profession which itself possesses a more clearly-marked management hierarchy than does the medical profession. Much nurse quality assurance has been introduced and run by nurse managers rather than (as in the case of medical audit) by nominal 'peers'.
- *Some* (not all) of the methods used make specific reference to the need to consult patients and take heed of their views and preferences.

Because of these differences we believe that, within our threefold taxonomy of quality, most of the activities nurses have been engaged in are essentially examples of the pursuit of *service quality*. That is, they are mainly driven from the 'provider' perspective but they focus on both physical/technical *and* psychosocial aspects of service delivery and are quite open to management influences and management concerns.

It may help briefly to describe one of the most widely-adopted systems, Nurse Monitor. Monitor is questionnaire-based, with a somewhat different instrument being used according to the patient dependency level ('minimal care', 'average care', 'above average care' and 'maximum care'); 80–150 questions will be asked of the care of any given patient, drawn from a total bank of 455 Monitor questions. Trained assessors (typically two per ward) administer the questionnaires. They cover four main dimensions: assessment and planning, physical care, non-physical care and evaluation. The following are examples:

- 'Is there a statement written within 24 hours of admission on the condition of the skin?' (Assessment and Planning).
- 'Is adequate equipment for oral hygiene available?' (Physical Care).
- 'Do the nursing staff call the patient by the name he prefers?' (Non-physical Care).
- 'Do records document the effect of the administration of 'as required' medication?' (Evaluation).

The questions are answered by the assessors after they have sought information from the records, the nurses, directly from the patient and by observation. Eventually an overall score is computed by awarding 1 for a 'yes' and 0 for a 'no' to each question. Thus the highest possible score would be a 'perfect' 100 per cent.

Monitor and most other systems for assessing nursing quality reflect characteristic features of contemporary nursing. On the one hand they are coloured by nursing's aspiration to the status of a fully-independent profession with distinctive scientific methods. Hence the emphasis on carefully tested questionnaires, trained assessors and applicability to 'the nursing process'. From this perspective 'quality' is a matter of achieving technical standards generated from within the profession. Thus it is possible, for example, for a nurse to score quite highly on Monitor while doing rather little to meet the patient's actual wants. What the nurse should do and say with the patient is defined by the profession, not by the patient.

On the other hand the subjective views of the patient do loom larger (especially in Qualpac) than in most medical audit. Nursing systems are also more likely than most medical audit to acknowledge and allow for the fact that health care is delivered not by one profession but by a wide variety of mutually dependent occupational groups. This contrast is most painfully obvious in Phaneuf audit where the first of the seven underlying nursing functions is identified as 'the application and execution of the physician's legal orders'. Indeed, to some extent the development of systems for nursing quality assessment may be seen as yet another in a long line of defences constructed by nurses to strengthen their powers of resistance to *ad hoc* interference in nursing activities by the medical profession. Nurse managers can now point to apparently scientific quality ratings as justification for organizing nursing care in *their* way. The reciprocal is that, with a few exceptions, nurses remain excluded from the medical domain. We remember the comment of one senior nurse, appointed Director of Standards, who ruefully observed that he was now responsible for all quality standard-setting in the district – except medical standards, over which he had no influence whatsoever.

However, the systematization of nursing quality can be a two-edged sword. In so far as measurement systems make nursing activities more transparent to middle and senior management, and in so far as they facilitate the definition of standard 'package of care' they may increase the scope for hierarchical control and the dominance of managerial over professional values. Systems which help defend nurses from medical 'interference' may also increase their vulnerability to managerial intervention (see also the discussion of nursing RM earlier in this chapter). Indeed the introduction of Monitor, Qualpac, etc. has been paralleled by the rapid growth of managerial analyses of nursing skill mix, driven primarily by a concern for the economical and efficient deployment of the NHS's most expensive single resource. For example, the computerized Excelcare system, piloted in West Dorset, is first and foremost an approach to measuring nursing outcomes. But it also leads to the definition of standard 'units of care' which can serve as a basis for workload allocation and costing.

Finally, we should correct any impression we may have given that all quality efforts in nursing have taken the form of elaborate systems imported from North America. Whilst these have certainly been important there have also been a vast number of local initiatives, often nurse-initiated, bearing quality labels of one kind or another. The variety here has been great: patient satisfaction surveys, the writing and distribution of patient handbooks, new signposts around hospital sites, improved complaints systems, more liberal visiting hours, creation of 'patients perceptions groups' and so on. A 1989 survey identified 1478 quality initiatives which were then underway in England and Wales, and nurses appeared to be involved in a majority of these.

The final topic for this section is Total Quality Management. During 1989–90 the Department of Health launched a funding programme aimed at supporting health authorities which submitted suitable proposals for implementing TQM schemes. The first round of this programme resulted in financial support being awarded to 17 demonstration sites, with further sites being added later.

The TQM programme was a managerially-led exercise which attempted to adapt a set of tools originally developed in private sector manufacturing for use in NHS settings. TQM has been variously defined, and there are rival approaches within it, but textbook formulation commonly include the following elements:

- A corporate approach to quality – usually marked by the production of an organization-wide plan which includes specific quality goals.
- Real commitment to and enthusiasm for quality improvement, from top management down to the 'front line'.
- A transcendence of departmental and disciplinary boundaries. Many quality improvement possibilities typically lie *across* such intra-organizational boundaries.
- A willingness to invest in training.
- A commitment to *continuous improvement*. TQM is seen as an on-going process, not a once-and-for-all setting of standards.
- An emphasis on avoiding 'mistakes'/defects *before* they happen, rather than correcting them retrospectively (and often expensively). This element of TQM is often referred to as 'getting it right first time'.

The ministerial press release at the launch of the TQM programme echoed the somewhat evangelical tone of much private sector TQM literature. TQM, it claimed:

> aims to harness the efforts of management and all staff in ensuring that every aspect of their work is directed towards the attainment of high quality. It puts the need of the patient at the centre of health service provision.

The last point is particularly important. The concept of quality which underlies TQM is not one of technically-defined excellence (though such excellence may well be an outcome of TQM) but rather quality as fitness for the purposes and needs of the service.

Thus, as the junior minister proclaimed at the launch: 'These initiatives will further develop services geared to the requirements of the patient'. Thus if, for example, most patients for a particular service want the service to be faster, while most of the doctors and nurses providing the service want it to be technically more sophisticated it should normally be speed rather than technical enhancement which takes priority.

Early experiences at the TQM demonstration sites do not yet offer a firm basis for assessing the ultimate potential of TQM within the NHS. They do, however, embody some ominous, if not unexpected warnings of difficulties ahead. An interim assessment by independent researchers indicated that several problems were common. First, evaluation of the projects was rendered extremely difficult because providers had no fixed quality benchmarks from which they had started. Thus it was frequently impossible to show how large or small an alleged quality improvement had been. Second, the regular and wholehearted participation of the medical profession was the exception rather than the rule. Perhaps connected to this was the finding that core medical activities were rarely the focus for early TQM efforts. The term 'Total' in NHS-style TQM was misleading. Third, inter-departmental boundaries often proved hard to dissolve. Blaming problems on 'them' continued as a popular pastime. Fourth, there was a degree of understandable confusion about how TQM was supposed to relate to all the other changes going on – medical and nursing audit, Resource Management, new information systems, contracting and so on. Again, TQM seemed in practice to be 'another thing to do' rather than something which was truly 'total' in the sense that it embraced and infused all other major organizational processes. Also the resources going into NHS TQM programmes appeared to be only a tenth of those devoted to parallel TQM 'installations' in, say, Post Office Counters or the Thames Water Company. On the other hand TQM was a useful banner under which local enthusiasms were being roused and particular improvements carried through. If it was not yet a catalyst for wholesale cultural change (as some of its private sector gurus claimed it should be) then it was at least a lever which could be seized to promote and accelerate piecemeal and incremental change, both in attitudes and practices.[26]

In drawing together our observations on quality assessment and assurance, it is evident that the NHS is currently bubbling with a mixed stew of 'quality' initiatives (we could have mentioned others such as the King's Fund accreditation scheme or the DoH's Waiting Lists Initiative). It is equally apparent that the pot is flavoured with all three of our notions of professionalism. Medical audit, for example, is heavily laced with the functional notion. The medical profession regulates itself through (in this case) peer review of the technical quality of its work. In doing this doctors are to be free from all outside interference, and can be trusted always to act in the best interests of their patients.

Yet medical audit also carries the less pleasant taste of professional self-interest. It has been set up in such a way that management is largely excluded and the patients totally excluded. Substandard practices can go unpunished (other than by a few stern words from colleagues) and those outside the charmed circle need never know. When (as happened in one teaching hospital we visited) obstetricians vigorously reject the very idea of including a representative of the midwives on their audit committee one suspects that inter-professional jealousies are more to the fore than the interests of patients.

The flavour of our third notion of professionalism is less obvious, but it is there all the same. Consider the diversity of ways in which the Government have approached the issue of maintaining and improving quality in the new circumstances of a provider market. How can one explain the simultaneous espousal within the same organization of a corporate, consumer-oriented doctrine such as TQM and a mono-professional, provider-focussed technique such as medical audit? This *could* be construed as the state tightening its grip on most groups of health care workers (including nurses) while continuing to allow the medical élite just enough autonomy to ensure that they, and not the politicians, continue to carry most of the responsibility for painful micro-rationing decisions on exactly which patients to treat. With resource management increasingly in place medical expenditures at directorate level are far more programmed and capped than during the first 40 years of the NHS, so what harm is there in allowing doctors a private playground for discretionary decisions? Meanwhile nurses and other health care professional and non-professional workers are subject to ever-more systematic work measurement and 'rationalization'. Managers are the Government's instruments in enforcing these new disciplines, and a mixture of short-term contracts and performance pay help ensure their loyalty to central policies. This is clearly not the only possible interpretation of the current state of play, but neither is it a plainly absurd one.

Given that elements of all three notions of professionalism may be present in the current quality maelstrom, what may be forecast for the medium term future ? First, there seems little sign of effective resistance to the continuing systematization of nursing. The nursing process is becoming steadily more transparent to and manipulable by managers, be they nurse managers or general managers. Dependency levels, skill mixes, quality standards – all are the subject of increasing measurement efforts and the age of the 'costed package' of nursing is already with us. It is hard to see how the nursing profession could resist this on-going trend, indeed many of its brightest and best actively support it.

Second, the medical profession has had considerable short term success in regaining control of the 'quality' of its product following the shock of *Working for Patients*. Yet the bastion of medical autonomy is far from invulnerable. Even the basic fact that all doctors are now *supposed* to do audit subtly enhances the position of management. Management is now entitled to ask whether audit is being conducted, how it is being conducted and whether everyone who should be is taking part. Furthermore, it is entitled to demand aggregate audit data, and may use – or may be obliged to use – this in negotiations over provider contracts. Although no new disciplinary procedures have yet been put in place managers are in a stronger position than they were to insist to leading consultants that the medical peer group informally disciplines its own members effectively. The profession may have drawn up the waggons round medical audit, but outside the circle managers have increasing control over – or at least intelligence about – the supplies going to the defenders of medical autonomy.

Third, we should consider the position of those who use the NHS. Are they now part of the quality game? Despite the heady rhetoric of the TQM gurus it is hard to see that patients and citizens have more than walk-on parts. The predominant conceptualizations of quality remain professional – as in medical or nursing audit – and where they are not professional they are mostly managerial. Patients are certainly consulted more often than in the past, but the consultations are usually on management's terms. Now they are frequently asked what they think of the services on offer, but seldom what services they would like to see on offer or how they themselves would define and assess quality. What is more they are asked for their opinions but they are in no way empowered to ensure that notice is taken of their views once expressed. TQM may be built around the notion of 'fitness for purpose' but the data collected on patients' *purposes* is still very thin. Ticking the boxes on a management-designed patient satisfaction questionnaire is a long way short of 'services geared to the requirements of patients'.

# 5

# CHANGING THE ENVIRONMENT

## INTRODUCTION

Under this heading we deal with two strategies whose common element is an attempt to control the larger *environment* in which professionals. Both strategies were entwined in the 1989 White Paper *Working for Patients*. The first is the creation of the 'purchaser/provider split' in health (and social) care. The second is the ostensible empowerment of NHS consumers. The theoretical connection here is that if an organization's external environment becomes more demanding than before, the influence of those responsible for managing the internal/external boundary (i.e. managers) is enhanced. Certainly if the *number* of managers is an indicator of their power *Working for Patients* marked a leap forward: between 1939 and 1991 the number of managers employed in the NHS regions increased by 7610 (while the number of nurses fell by 3450).[1]

## THE PURCHASER/PROVIDER SPLIT

Tracing the history of ideas is not an easy matter, and we are not able to identify with any confidence the original source of the notion of a separation between what have subsequently been termed the 'purchasing' and 'providing' functions[2] within a *publicly-funded* health service. These functions have been distinguished as follows (Harrison 1991):

> Within monolithic welfare state institutions, including, in Britain [old style] District Health Authorities and local

authority social services departments, two distinct functions can be discerned analytically. One role or function is relatively straightforward; the *provider* role entails the ownership of hospitals and other care institutions, the employment of direct health care staff such as doctors and nurses, and the provision of health and related services directly to the patient or client. Perhaps more difficult to discern is the other, *purchaser* role, that is, the identification of needs and priorities within and between patient or population groups, and the subsequent direction of financial resources toward services that will meet those needs and priorities.

There seems little doubt, however, that part of the responsibility for popularizing the notion of the split can be allocated to Professor Alain Enthoven, an economist and former US government official. Invited to the UK in the mid-1980s, Enthoven produced an outline prescription for an NHS 'internal market'.[3] In this model, District Health Authorities (DHAs) would receive funds for the health care of their *resident* population, but be free to choose for themselves the balance between the amount of care the District directly provided, and the amount it purchased from other DHAs. In Enthoven's view, this would both provide an incentive for the more efficient utilization of beds and other resources (because funds would follow the patient to the providing institution), and provide a counter-weight to what he regarded as the excessive influence of consultant medical staff (because they would need to attract patients in order to obtain resources for their service).

In the event, the model subsequently introduced in the UK as a result of the White Paper *Working for Patients* was somewhat different.[4] It is sketched out in Figure 5.1, which indicates financial flows (not lines of authority) based on resident populations of districts. DHAs act as *purchasers* of care for their residents, being responsible for identifying and prioritizing local needs, entering into contracts[5] with providers, and monitoring the results. There are four types of provider institution with whom a DHA may contract: the private sector, the DHA's own institution, another DHA's own institution (these are termed 'directly-managed units' or DMUs) and NHS Trusts. These last institutions have been allowed by the Government to leave DHA control and become 'self-governing'.[6] The crucial point is that providers are almost entirely dependent for revenue on contracts to treat patients. The

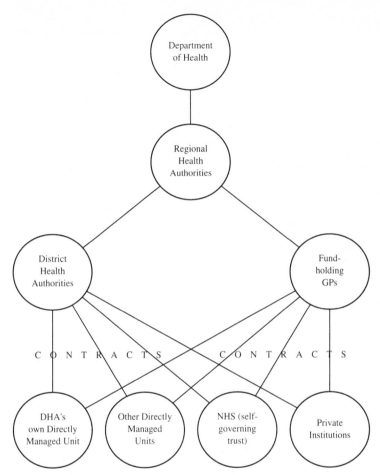

**Figure 5.1**    The purchaser/provider split in English health care

*Source:* Adapted from S. Harrison, D.J. Hunter and C. Pollitt (1990) *The Dynamics of British Health Policy.* Unwin Hyman, London.

pressure from purchasers can be – and has been – increased by the formation of purchasing consortia or mergers of DHAs, or even of DHAs and FHSAs.

It will be evident that the above scheme of things is, in one sense, *more radical* than Enthoven's proposals; although the latter certainly included the *concept* of the purchaser/provider split, the degree of organizational separation entailed in the creation of NHS Trusts was not. It is clear, however, that Enthoven would have liked to be more radical had he felt it politically feasible to be so. Concluding his prescription, he observed (Enthoven 1985a):

> From an economic point of view, the main defect in this model is that it still lacks powerful incentives for District Managers to make their decisions . . . in the face of . . . pressures to favour inside suppliers in the interests of keeping peace in the family . . . I believe that the internal market model offers substantial improvement over the present NHS structure. But I wouldn't promise the full benefits of the kind of competing [health maintenance organization] scheme we are developing in the United States. When all of the alternatives have been considered, it becomes apparent that there is nothing like a competitive market to motivate and economy of service.

The reader will have noted that we have not yet mentioned the fundholding GPs which appear in Figure 5.1. In fact, the fundholding practice is an arrangement which draws very obviously on the American health maintenance organization (HMO) notion mentioned by Enthoven.[7] The UK version of this deducts elements from the funding of DHAs and allocates them directly to volunteer GPs; the latter are then able to enter into their own contractual arrangements with providers of secondary and community care.[8] Thus fundholding GPs become a second category of purchaser, alongside DHAs.

In concentrating upon Enthoven and the UK, however, there is a danger of ignoring developments elsewhere, for the purchaser/provider split seems very much to be the proverbial 'idea whose time has come'.[9] An increasing number of European countries are incorporating the split into redesigns of their health services.[10] However, there are several, rather different, approaches, which we have summarized in Figure 5.2. The horizontal dimension represents the provider function; it distinguishes between an arrangement in which hospitals and other care organizations are wholly publicly owned, and those in which privately owned institutions are permitted to participate. The *Working for Patients* scheme is, of course, a *mixed* market, since privately owned organizations are free to bid for DHA and GP fundholder contracts.

The vertical dimension of Figure 5.2 denotes the purchasing function. It distinguishes between a market proper, in which the

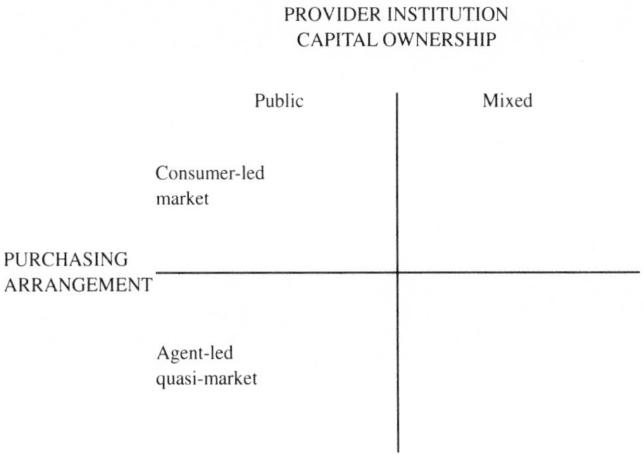

PROVIDER INSTITUTION
CAPITAL OWNERSHIP

|  | Public | Mixed |
|---|---|---|
| Consumer-led market | | |
| PURCHASING ARRANGEMENT | | |
| Agent-led quasi-market | | |

**Figure 5.2** A typology of approaches to the purchaser/provider split in secondary health care

*Source:* Adapted from R.B. Saltman, S. Harrison and C. von Otter (1991) 'Designing competition for publicly funded health system.' In D.J. Hunter (ed.), *Paradoxes of Competition for Health*. Nuffield Institute for Health Services Studies, Leeds.

patient/consumer exercises choice of provider (even if not paying out of pocket), and a quasi-market in which choice is exercised by someone else (an *agent*), either a managerial organization (such as, in the UK, a DHA) or a primary care doctor (the HMO/GP fundholding model).[11] The reformed NHS is therefore an agent-led mixed market (bottom right-hand cell).

But how does all this add up to a strategy for controlling health professionals in the UK? Though it is difficult to find a full statement of the argument, it seems to run along the following lines:

● The continued conflation of purchaser and provider functions within a monolithic health care or social care organization creates a service which is *producer-oriented*. First, there are no incentives to efficiency (since more patients/clients will not produce more money) and, second, there are no incentives to respond to other than *professional* definitions of what patients need (since need identification, provision of services, and judgements about performance are all contained within one set of actors). This view of a health care organization as 'judge and jury in its own court' is an amalgam of the second (occupational control) view of professionalism which we discussed in Chapter 1 and what is often termed 'public choice theory'.[12]

● A purchaser/provider split which is reinforced by a commensurate organizational split (e.g. the creation of NHS Trusts) allows market or quasi-market competition to occur, thereby promoting efficiency. Professionals will have to support the provider organization in its drive to compete, in order to ensure its survival and their jobs.

● The purchaser/provider split allows other judgements of need to compete with, or take precedence over, professional judgements. Just *whose* is this 'other' judgement is determined by the location of a particular health system within Figure 5.2; in the upper half, it would be the consumer's judgement, whereas in the lower half (including the UK case) it would be the manager or GP.

The argument thus far prompts a question: why did the Thatcher Government plump for a quasi-market rather than simply a market? Our answer is that the quasi-market allows some of the possibilities of control provided by a hierarchy to be added to the pressures created by the market. The DHA *purchasers* can still be controlled by a hierarchical line of authority that runs directly from the Secretary of State. Their purchasing budgets can be cash limited and their key staff appointed and (where necessary) dismissed. Yet at the same time the *providers* are obliged to compete and therefore (according to the theory) in the financial circumstances which were outlined in Chapter 2, retaining such control is a matter of some importance to a UK government. It is not surprising therefore that pains were taken to ensure that sufficient provider units 'volunteered' themselves as NHS Trusts. The new organizational status was attractive to managers, offering them enhanced freedom of operation and increased material rewards. The results of local ballots amongst consultants, often producing large majorities against seeking Trust status, were ignored. Box 5.1 contains extracts from a detailed account of how one mental health unit in the north of England became one of the first group of Trusts to be created.

It is, of course, early days to reach confident judgements about the effect of the purchaser/provider split on managerial control over health professionals. But *some* evidence is available, and the assessment which follows is therefore based on a (hopefully) judicious blending of this evidence with informed speculation.

**Box 5.1** Applying for trust status: overcoming the opposition

The letter [from the mental health unit] expressing an interest in Trust status stated that it had a substantial body of support within the unit . . . In fact, none of the formal managerial bodies or professional advisory groups . . . had been consulted over, much less assented to, this expression . . . Two [general managers] went to region to discuss the expression of interest. With them, they took a letter from the United Medical Representative which recorded the opposition of all but one consultant to the expression. This letter . . . was not regarded as important by regional officers.

. . . opposition took two . . . forms. The first was the attempt to create mass resistance under the banner of '[Mental Health Unit] Opposition to the White Paper Campaign' . . . with its own Bulletin and regular meetings . . . The second method of resistance was through the [multidisciplinary management teams] . . . and it was clear that . . . there was a clear majority of [team] members opposed to the expression of interest . . .

In fact, the threat turned out to be transient. The UGM focused his political skill and will on a number of key consultants, evey flying in two American professors to discuss the impact of contracting . . . The attempted resistance through [management teams] was either ignored or deflected by [general managers] usually under the guise of advising [them] to await further information . . .

The decision whether or not to pursue an application for NHS Trust status was the single most important and controversial one that had faced the unit since the arrival of the [unit general manager]. It is, therefore, an excellent indicator of where the power lay in the decision making process within the unit . . . The conclusion is that the power resided with the [managers] and that this reflected the *increasing consolidation of power in the system of personal formal authority at the expense of the system of expertise [emphasis added]*.

*Source:* E. Peck (1991) 'Power in the National Health Service: a case study of a unit considering NHS Trust status', *Health Services Management Research*, 4(2): 128–9.

**Box 5.2**   Bottomley rejects nurses' plea to ban gagging clauses

*David Brindle, Social Services Correspondent*

The Health Secretary, Virginia Bottomley, yesterday refused to outlaw 'gagging' clauses in health workers' contracts after nursing leaders claimed there was a climate of fear in the service.

Mrs Bottomley said that while nurses had a duty to take up issues of concern, it was reasonable for employers to expect them to do so without running to the press.

The Royal College of Nursing released a report at its annual congress in Blackpool yesterday showing that more than 100 nurses had contacted a 'whistle-blow' service set up to enable them to raise concerns without being identified.

Christine Hancock, the college general secretary, said gagging clauses were symptomatic of a 'macho' culture taking root among National Health Service managers.

'Gagging clauses seem to be an example of public service managers imitating what they believe to be a business culture. In contrast, most successful businesses recognise that you cannot build a good, corporate image on top of underlying problems over staffing and resources.'

The college's report precedes the broadcast tonight on BBC2 of a documentary on Graham Pink, the nurse sacked after campaigning for more staff on his wards for elderly patients at Stepping Hill hospital, Stockport. Mr Pink sprang to prominence after the Guardian published extracts of his correspondence on conditions on his wards. He has launched a public appeal for £50 000 to enable him to contest his dismissal at an industrial tribunal.

The college report monitors the first 10 months of the whistle-blow service, during which time many other nurses are said to have raised concerns openly or directly with the college.

One of those who used the service wrote: 'I did my early shift from 7am and the staff who came on in the afternoon were not trained or experienced enough to give out the medication. I worked an extra three or four hours to try to help the other staff who were totally stretched and under pressure. In the end, I left the ward in tears, too tired to do any more and afraid of what would happen to the patients later.'

A second nurse wrote: 'Anyone who attempts to rectify the situation by approaching management is labelled a trouble-maker.'

Ms Hancock said: 'Commonly, nurses perceive that managers have absorbed the culture of competition and commercial confidence and forgotten that they are managing an accountable public service.'

While nurses should not go to the press at the first sign of difficulty, they had to be free to voice their concerns and should have a legal right to do so without recrimination.

Mrs Bottomley told reporters at the conference: 'Nurses not only have a responsibility, they have a duty to take up situations where they are worried about professional care of patients. I want to work to make that clear to nurses, to doctors and to managers, but I don't think we have reached the stage of looking at legislation.'

Pressed on the acceptability of gagging clauses, she said: 'It's reasonable for employers to expect their staff first of all to raise points of concern with the management.'

*Whistleblow: Nurses Speak Out; RCN, 20 Cavendish Square, London W1M 0AB; free.*

Source: *The Guardian*, 28 April 1992. © *The Guardian*.

Our first observation is that the change in the organizational environment brought about by the purchaser/provider split adds a degree of 'bite' to some of the earlier developments which we discussed in Chapters 3 and 4. In particular, the split increases the pressure to define and cost services, thereby making professional activities (in all the health professions) increasingly transparent to managers. Let us take Resource Management (RM) as an example.

At risk of oversimplification one might say that, in the NHS quasi-market, the chief executive of a provider hospital has two main problems in his or her organizational life. One is to obtain business for the institution; without contracts to treat patients, it will have few or no resources. The other is to deliver on those contracts. It is easy to see that RM is a crucial component of both processes. Without it (or something like it), it is difficult to see how realistic costs can be calculated and appropriate prices quoted.[13] Equally, since the manager is not personally in a position to provide services to fulfil contracts, but can only do so via health professionals, some method of setting and controlling workloads and budgets is vital.

It is unnecessary for us to do more than list other examples of the same principle at work. For instance, cost pressures add to the necessity for the various forms of controls over (especially) nurse staffing levels which we discussed in Chapter 3. The fact that contracts largely define patient cases in terms of medical specialty strengthens the case for the development of forms of hospital organization based on clinical directorates or similar structures. And the need to defend institutions against allegations of 'low price/low quality' provides a strong rationale for the further application of audit and quality assurance systems of the kinds discussed in Chapter 4. Finally, the ostensibly competitive situation of providers can be used to justify attempts to discipline professional staff for speaking out in the face of what the latter perceive as inadequate services for patients. Box 5.2 gives one example of this, though it is by no means only nurses who have been threatened in this way.[14] Eventually ministers intervened with a compromise solution: 'gagging' clauses were not to be outlawed but complaint channels were to be provided that would reach all the way up the management hierarchy to the NHS Chief Executive.[15]

The above observations apply to all health professionals. Our second set is applicable more specifically to doctors. The purchaser/provider split has served to justify a level of managerial involvement in what were previously 'no go' areas. Box 5.3 is a quotation from a report of research carried out during the first year of the NHS quasi-market. Note how the change in organizational environment appears to create new leverage for both purchaser *and* provider managers over medical professionals.[16] In general, so far as the relationships between doctors and managers are concerned (Harrison *et al.* 1992), the purchaser/provider split

> . . . appears to mark a genuine watershed. It puts several additional levers of power and persuasion into managers

---

**Box 5.3** Using the purchaser/provider split to influence doctors

So far as 'quality' is concerned, in three authorities DHA officers and GPs had identified a number of areas in which providers performance was deficient. These included ophthalmic waiting times, attitudes of consultant obstetricians to patients, orthopaedic outcomes and direct access by GPs to physiotherapy services. As a result, these DHAs would consider threatening to move contracts elsewhere, though they would not place contracts with different providers without giving existing ones the opportunity to improve their performance in 1992–93. This action was being contemplated in one case because the DHA felt it was necessary to be seen to be responsive to GP opinions; it is perhaps significant that the authority was one with an above average – and increasing – penetration of GP fundholding. Although this DHA was being careful not to issue direct threats since it feared a destructive spiral of deteriorating relationships, consultants here and elsewhere were reported to be aware of the possibility of losing their services under the new arrangements and it was anticipated that this would lead to peer group pressure being applied to improve quality where this was necessary. The potential shift in the balance of influence from consultants towards purchasers and GPs had also been appreciated by provider managers who saw the external threat to remove contracts as a source of additional leverage for them to apply on consultants.

*Source:* S. Harrison and G. Wistow (1992) 'The purchaser/provider split in English health care: towards explicit rationing?', *Policy and Politics*, 20(2).

---

hands, in a way which Griffiths . . . did not. These are not overwhelming powers, and we predict no spectacular collapse of the medical citadel. Even if used with skill and determination it would probably take some years before a general manager could hope to exert a regular, systematic and substantial influence on clinical workloads, clinical quality or clinical priorities. In many cases we imagine individual general managers will lack either the skill or the determination – most likely the latter, in the light of the rest of their overloaded agendas. Nevertheless, for the first time the basis for trimming the variance of local medical practice is there, and no doubt some will try to use it.

Meanwhile the fortunes of managers as a group have certainly waxed considerably over the last decade. The 'diplomat' model of the administrator . . . is now almost dead.

Before leaving the issue of the purchaser/provider split there are two further consequences – or at least possible consequences – of note. The first of these is that it is not only the relations between managers and professionals which are affected by the new arrangements – intra-professional relations may also undergo change. Members of the same profession may find it harder than formerly to make common cause because they are now on opposite sides of a quasi-market relationship. One may work for a purchaser, another for a provider. Or they may work for competing providers in the same locality. All this further reduces the probability of successful professional resistance to management. Previous differences in intra-professional *status* may also be transformed by the advent of the purchaser/provider split. Perhaps the most notable example of this is the enhanced influence of budget-holding GP practices vis-à-vis hospital-based consultants. For the first time such GPs are now in a position to 'take their business elsewhere' *and exact a financial penalty on the providing hospital.*[17] This assumes, however, that consultants continue to be what they usually are at present – salaried employees of a particular provider, unable much to move their own services around from one provider to another. If we relax this assumption – as we do in Chapter 6 – the picture begins to change again. The second and final observation is that, although the NHS market is frequently referred to as a 'provider market', implying that it is only the *providers* who compete, it is possible that *purchaser* competition could also develop. To a limited extent this is already visible in cases where individual GP budgetholders drive more advantageous deals with providers than the local DHA or consortium. Although the idea of purchaser competition is currently politically sensitive (and actual examples are therefore usually covert) it would represent a further extension of the market logic of which the Conservative administration is so obviously fond.

It could be explicitly organized within a framework of rules designed to reward those purchasers who secured best value for money for their resident populations. However, this is largely speculative, and further discussion will therefore be deferred until Chapter 6.

## EMPOWERING THE CONSUMER?

Why should consumer empowerment and currently fashionable ideas about increasing patient choice restrict the autonomy of professionals? One obvious way in which this could happen would be if the enlargement of patient choice was obtained by a diminution of professional choice, i.e. if decisions of a type that had formerly been taken *for* the patient by the professional were henceforth taken by the patient for him or herself. In this way a policy of consumer empowerment, *even if it had not been embarked upon with the express intention of reducing professional autonomy*, could end up having that effect.

However, a direct transfer of decisional power is not the only possibility. The network of relationships is more complex, and allow for a number of other possibilities. For example:

● That consumers are given increased power only over issues in which professionals have little interest, such as waiting-room facilities, the interior decoration of wards or the range of food on offer.
● That increased consumer power impacts on *managerial* discretion as much as on professional autonomy. This could happen if consumers were given greater influence/choice in respect of essentially administrative arrangements such as appointments or over policy issues such as resource allocation which have previously been firmly in the grip of senior managers.
● That increased consumer power *does* infringe on the autonomy of professional groups, but in a very uneven way. This would happen if the less powerful professions were obliged to accept greater consumer choice in respect of their activities but the more powerful ones – medicine in particular – were still able to preserve their autonomy more or less unscathed.

In practice, as we shall see, the phenomenon of 'consumerism' is so pervasive, and the internal divisions of the NHS so complex, that

**Box 5.4**   The impact of the Griffiths changes on consumer orientation

The traditional NHS model depended on rationing output to a passive patient population. For some time, the reality of more informed and critical patient population has created problems for NHS managers and clinicians. While consumerism was placed centre stage by the White Paper, *Working for Patients*, in theory Griffiths had already injected a degree of consumer orientation upon which to build. Our study uncovered a great deal of cynicism regarding things like 'window-dressing', 'charm school training' and *ad hoc* market research. For a more optimistic view see Chantler's account of events at Guy's Hospital (Chantler 1988: 10–11). The Templeton College team assert that DGMs have been attracted to versions of consumerism which do not necessitate their entering the clinical domain. Our own study revealed 'quality' and consumerism to be concepts pigeon-holed with a particular post in the organization (usually held by a senior nurse) rather than something which had entered the mainstream of organizational culture. Strong and Robinson's respondents reacted cynically to the tendency for DGMs to off-load the consumer-relations job into the domain of nurse managers. They quote a District Medical Officer who (unusually) also held the post of Director of Quality (Strong and Robinson 1990):

> some of the nurses and quality terrify me! . . . I've been really shocked by some of the ones I've met. They haven't a clue. They thought it was all about dealing with patients' complaints . . . some of the ones I've met think the idea is to get quality printed on T-shirts! . . . To give it to nurses just sets up the whole problem all over again.

Strong and Robinson conclude that consumer orientation, and in particular the emphasis on quality, is really no more than a political gesture with little real meaning. While some initiatives have been worthwhile, we believe that the evidence for the period 1985 to 1990 indicates that the context in which general management was implemented militated against an imaginative and purposeful consumer orientation emerging in the NHS.

*Source:* S. Harrison, D.J. Hunter, G. Marnoch and C. Pollitt (1992) *Just Managing: Power and Culture in the NHS*, 94–5. Macmillan, London.
(Full references for primary quotations are to be found in the Bibliography.)

there is some evidence of *all* these different kinds of impact occurring at least somewhere.

First, we need to revisit the 1983 Griffiths report which recommended the introduction of general management. One of Griffiths' arguments was that insufficient attention was paid to meeting users' expectations of the service. The Griffiths prescription, however, was rather vague: managers should pay more attention to consumer opinion. Perhaps not surprisingly, therefore, there seems to have been little substantive result. Box 5.4 sums up the findings of several post-Griffiths research studies on the topic.

*Working for Patients* was more ambitious. According to the Department of Health, Welsh Office, Northern Ireland Central Office and Scottish Office (1989: 3), one of its two stated objectives was

> . . . to give patients, wherever they live in the UK better health care and *greater choice of the services available.* (emphasis added)

There were three main means by which consumer influence was to be attained: changes in the GP contract and associated regulations, the new role of DHAs as purchasing authorities, and the creation of GP fundholding. We discuss each of these in turn.

First, a number of important changes were made to the GP contract, which had the effect of placing increased financial importance on variable payments related to list size rather than fixed ones such as practice allowances. Thus, capitation fees[18] were to increase in importance from a little over 40 per cent to some 60 per cent of the average GP's income. Coupled with a change in the regulations which abolished the need for a patient to seek his or her present GP's approval before registering with a different practice and which required practice information leaflets, this would theoretically make the GP more keen to respond to patient preferences in order not to lose registrants, and thereby income. Given the apparently very high level of public satisfaction with GPs,[19] and the lack of accessible alternative practices in many areas, it is difficult to envisage a shift of influence towards patients, though it might perhaps create a degree of insecurity for the GP. Second, we consider the establishment of DHAs as purchasing authorities in the context of the purchaser/provider split. The particular approach to the purchaser/provider split adopted in the UK does not empower consumers directly but rather empowers their *agents* (Figure

**Box 5.5**   DHA purchasers and the public

. . . all of our respondents were conscious that it was important to achieve a higher level of contact between purchasers and the public, though approaches to this varied. Our most proactive and assertive purchasing authority had also been the most active in seeking out public opinion. Thus, it had circulated 2500 copies of its draft health plan, together with a supporting questionnaire, to organizations within its area. A 10 per cent response had been achieved with further replies expected through the local authority. Preliminary results were seen to be threatening to the main provider unit because they suggested that community rather than hospital-based care for elderly people was emerging as a priority. A marketing firm had also been commissioned both to carry out a postal questionnaire, with follow-up interviews, of general practitioners and also to conduct interviews with over a thousand local people. Moreover the authority was planning to stimulate public debate by the publication of an adversarial dialogue between proponents and opponents of the funding of IVF. Another authority was in the process of establishing, in conjunction with its FHSA, a standing panel of a similar number of local residents to be used as a regular sounding board for the identification of needs and priorities.

A third authority was more cautious about consulting the public and appeared to be restricting itself to the provision of more information to local people rather than obtaining information from them. One of our respondents in this authority suggested that public surveys ran the risk of creating too high public expectations and that 'the public are not well enough educated to make choices about health care'. Accepting that non-executive members of the DHA did not represent the public (and that business oriented non-executives were not appropriate to the purchasing role), the respondent envisaged using GPs as proxies for public opinion. Despite professions of the importance of consumer input as a legitimating force in a service without a local democratic element, none of our authorities had yet found it easy to work with their Community Health Council, asserting either or both that the CHC was 'too political' or 'still obsessed with provider issues'. In one case it seemed possible that the removal of local authority councillors from DHAs had led to the use of the CHC for party political purposes.

*Source:* S. Harrison and G. Wistow (1992) 'The purchaser/provider split in English health care: towards explicit rationing?', *Policy and Politics*, 20(2).

5.2). In the case of DHA purchasers, the agents are *managers*, and this form of organization therefore represents a challenge to the second of the three models of professionalism that we introduced in Chapter 1. One might say that this empowerment of managers *in the name of* consumers has the effect – intentionally or otherwise – of undermining the legitimacy of the claims of health professionals to 'know' what the consumer wants and needs. At the same time, it could enhance the legitimacy of managerial decisions by linking them with the supposition that managers act on behalf of consumers.

In practice, however, it remains an open question as to how far DHA purchasers seek to base their decisions on public opinion. Available evidence is not yet substantial, given that the purchaser/provider split has been in operation for only a few months. A 1992 national survey of District General Managers concluded that, in the placing of contracts, the views of local residents, whether expressed through the CHC or latterly through the results of surveys, remained of low importance.[20] Box 5.5 summarizes the results of one more detailed local study. From Box 5.5 we can see a variety of approaches, some quite elaborate, to the (genuine) problem of incorporating public opinion into managerial decisions. These are being further developed by a number of purchasing authorities under the rubric of 'locality purchasing'. Nevertheless, it is quite clear that what is happening is precisely such incorporation, rather than any direct 'reading off' of consumer preferences. By now, readers may be asking themselves whether such a process might not represent a challenge to the third of the approaches to professionalism that we outlined in Chapter 1: the one which portrays professional autonomy as a rationing device.

On the face of it there is indeed such a challenge. Indeed, it would appear that NHS managers and the Government would actually be *disadvantaged* by it, since previously implicit rationing decisions would become painfully explicit. So far, however, although there have been debates and occasional attempts to investigate the feasibility of explicit rationing,[21] the new purchasing authorities have succeeded in maintaining an implicit approach. Just how this has been achieved is exemplified in Box 5.6, again drawn from an early study of DHA purchasing.

Despite managerial authority to make purchasing decisions, the awkward areas have been largely left with doctors, through the device of 'low priority' lists. Once again the effect is to endow DHA

---

**Box 5.6**    Rationing by NHS purchasing authorities: just how explicit?

[Another] development was the consideration being given to the level of funding for 'low priority treatments'. One authority was faced with a provider unit developing expensive procedures in the expectation that they would be purchased by the DHA. However, the latter had already announced its decision not to purchase one of them (IVF, largely on grounds of its perceived ineffectiveness). In addition, the DHA's officers were considering recommending that the authority cut or abandon a number of other services (for example, rhinoplasty and breast surgery for cosmetic purposes, all removals of tattoos and warts, and varicose vein surgery). It was possible the authority would decide that such procedures should not be available at all. Other authorities did not envisage blanket refusals to provide such treatments but anticipated agreeing to purchase only very limited numbers each year in specified circumstances (for example, tattoo removal in cases of psychological distress). In all cases, the lists of 'low priority' treatments had been drawn up in consultation with public health physicians, *though it was largely expected that it would be the hospital consultants (i.e. the providers) who would act as the 'gatekeeper' of access.*

*Source:* S. Harrison and G. Wistow (1992) 'The purchaser/provider split in English health care: towards explicit rationing?', *Policy and Politics*, 20(2).

---

managers with the legitimacy of consumer empowerment whilst leaving a good deal of substantive practice unchanged.

Finally, we discuss GP fundholding. Under this arrangement, GPs, rather than DHA managers, act as purchasing agents for a defined range of secondary and tertiary care services. Whilst, as with the new contract for all GPs (see above), this cannot be regarded as a major empowerment of consumers, it does not at first sight appear to represent managerial control, but rather a shift between different sections of the medical profession. It can, however, be seen as an opportunity for increased managerial control, in two ways.

---

**Box 5.7** GPs offered pain-free purchasing

GPs will be free to 'purchase' services for their patients without the administrative burden of fund management, under a new initiative developed by Bath health authority.

The scheme could head off the potential threat to coherent healthcare planning by transferring increasingly large chunks of HA cash to GP fundholders.

Under the scheme – Practice Sensitive Purchasing – GPs are given a notional budget by the HA to 'buy' services for their patients.

Individual practice needs are then built into major contracts drawn up with providers by the HA, which retains the financial and organizational responsibility for contracting.

District general manager Andrew Wall said the project would give GPs the freedoms available to fundholders with none of the bureaucracy.

'Fundholders and provider units could be dealing with hundreds of contracts. Under this scheme the HA acts as a purchasing agent, reducing paperwork,' he said.

The project would also accommodate fundholders by giving them indicative budgets for services not covered by fundholder budgets.

Five pilot practices have been set up, and a further 49 out of 64 practices in the HA have expressed an interest in the scheme.

*Source: Health Service Journal* (14 May 1992: 30).

---

One way is fairly clear: because GP fundholders have to operate within a negotiated budget they are, in effect, being required to adopt managerial practices and perhaps also managerial values. GP fundholding can therefore be seen as analogous to RM for hospital doctors: part of a strategy of incorporation (see Chapter 4).

Another way in which GP fundholding could be seen as an opportunity for managerial control is more speculative because it entails a longer-term analysis. Briefly, the analysis is as follows. In the longer-term, DHA purchasing and GP fundholding cannot co-exist in their present form. This is because, if fundholding were to be extended to all GPs, the latter would be responsible in total for some 35 per cent of NHS expenditure; moreover, this would include a good deal of the most clearly discretionary (i.e. non-acute in the clinical sense) expenditure.[22] The ostensible role of purchasing authorities in identifying health care needs and priorities would thereby be greatly undermined. Most DHA expenditure would be non-discretionary. One way in which continued co-existence could be contrived would be for DHA purchasers gradually to take over elements of GP fundholder control. Initially, this would be a supportive and advisory role, but could develop into the situation where fundholders held workload-related budgets in the same way as hospital doctors.

There is already a discernible trend towards the eventual amalgamation of DHAs and Family Health Services Authorities (which hold GP contracts).[23] If such combined purchasers were the source of GP funds (rather than, as at present, RHAs), the dominant position of the *managerial*, rather than the professional, purchasing agent would be confirmed. Box 5.7 confirms that we are not the first people to be thinking in such terms.

We can now return to reconsider the different possible impacts of consumer empowerment which we identified at the beginning of this section. It would be wise to remind ourselves at the outset that the NHS has traditionally been a very paternalistic organization, and that 'consumerism' is still a recent implant. It may or may not flourish. If predicting the longer term effects of the purchaser/provider split is difficult forecasting the impacts of consumerism is almost impossible. Even generalizing about the present is hazardous, but our interpretation, at the time of writing, would run something like this:

- There has certainly been an upsurge of *talk* about consumers/patients since the 1989 *Working for Patients* White Paper.
- There have also been numerous local initiatives which are partly or wholly consumerist in intent.
- Relatively few of these seem to have intruded on the autonomy of the medical profession.
- Many have concerned the 'hotel' aspects of hospitalization, or, in other health care settings, have concentrated on appearances ('decor'), administrative procedures (especially appointments systems and visiting rules) and/or the provision of information (brochures, leaflets).

- Such changes do increase patient convenience, comfort, information and choice. They also oblige nurses, receptionists and some managers (particularly the junior ones) to 'change their ways'.
- On the whole, however, the impact of changes of this kind of senior management and on consultants has been limited. Consumers have not yet been allowed into the 'heartlands' of the power of these two groups, which are (respectively) resource allocation between services (managers) and diagnosis, referral and treatment (consultants).

A crucial area to watch will be the formulation and monitoring of standards. As explicit standards become more and more common (and are built into contracts) will consumers have a direct input into their specification, their status (mandatory? guidelines? optional?) and their monitoring?[24]

One interesting recent example was the inclusion in the Government's *Patient's Charter* of a standard that no-one should have to wait more than two years for a surgical operation. Nominally this was very much a consumerist standard, but what were its actual origins and consequences? First, it was not the product of any systematic consultation with patients or patients-to-be. Instead, like most of the other ingredients of the various documents issued under the *Citizen's Charter* it was something that Whitehall decided would be both feasible and popular. It conferred no new legal right but was rather a Government-fostered expectation. Central government then proceeded to insist that all health authorities pursued the elimination of waits of longer than two years. Effort and resources were diverted from other activities to try to satisfy this Government demand (a demand which was expressed with particular vigour as the 1992 General Election approached). The Government fully utilized its hierarchy of command via the NHS Management Executive region–district spine of general managers to ensure that this issue was thrust to the top of local agendas. The result was that a reduction in very long waits was indeed achieved. However, it seems very likely that in some cases this was accomplished at the cost of (unpublished) increases in the waiting times in the under-one-year category (i.e. a lot of shorter waits were marginally increased).[25]

Naturally, managers claim credit for 'successes' such as these. But whether consumerism will become an effective instrument for increasing managerial legitimacy relative to medical or nursing legitimacy is far from clear. Surveys continue to show that the public invest much higher levels of trust in doctors or nurses than managers. Professionals, too, can claim credit for any improvements which occur (and are probably more likely to be believed). They have their own very direct relationships with 'consumers' and, under pressure from managers and politicians, are certainly shrewd enough to cultivate patient loyalties. Nor, finally, can the activities of the consumers themselves be precisely controlled and predicted – whether by managers or professionals. Consumerism in the NHS is, as we said, fairly new. To what extent consumers will remain content with the rather limited role allocated to them by *Working for Patients* remains to be seen.

# 6

# THE FUTURE OF MANAGERIAL AND PROFESSIONAL WORK IN THE NHS

Some of the general points which emerge from the preceding five chapters are fairly obvious, others more subtle. We will take the obvious ones first. Most of the changes we have examined include some loss of autonomy for the individual health care professional. Compared with 20 – or even 10 – years ago the average professional's work is nowadays much more likely to be costed, audited, used as an input for performance indicators, subjected to explicit budgetary or workload ceilings (possibly embodied in a contract or service agreement) and/or included within the scope of patient satisfaction surveys. In addition to these largely or partly managerial controls, individual clinical decision-making may well have to take account of a multiplying number of guidelines or protocols laid down by professional bodies at national level.

In these senses, then, the previous conception of individualistic professionalism has been progressively replaced. In the 'old days' the NHS hospital could sometimes seem to exist *for* the doctors, rather than the other way round.[1] Pre-Griffiths administrators saw their role as one of *facilitating* the work of doctors and nurses, not controlling or directing them. However, the contemporary ethos is much more one of the professional as a member of a team, and beyond that, of an employing organization. The presumption is that the individual professional will be subject to the rules, plans and priorities of that organization (as well, perhaps, as the increasingly codified guidelines of the profession itself).

Meanwhile, of course, the powers of management have waxed formidably. From 1984 to 1989 general managers were put in place

and were immediately able to exert increased control over the
professions allied to medicine and over nurses. The medical profession itself proved less amenable to control by general managers,
but the 1990s have seen even their autonomy increasingly hedged
about by external factors (the purchaser/provider split and the
threat of competition) and internal controls (a more performance-
oriented contract for GPs imposed in 1990; as-good-as-mandatory
medical audit; new and more detailed local job descriptions for
consultants, etc.). And all the time the refinement of increasingly
sophisticated information systems have made the amounts and
types of nursing and medical work which is actually carried out
more and more transparent to the managers of provider units. Some
commentators have described these developments in terms of a
decline in relationships based principally on trust and a correspond-
ing increase in the measuring and monitoring of performance. It
seems clear that this changing relationship has as yet some way to
go. In particular, and despite some difficulties that we identified in
Chapter 5, we expect to see clinical decision-making increasingly
governed by locally determined diagnostic and treatment protocols,
based in part upon the effectiveness literature, and in part upon
local agreements between GPs, purchasers, and providers.[2]

Is the conclusion, then, that the 'future of work and organization
in the NHS' (our subtitle) is simply one of ever-growing management dominance in which professionals can at best look forward to a
future as well-paid workers within a series of tightly-managed
provider units, effectively shorn of most of their autonomy but still
permitted the symbols of their élite status in terms of titles and
regalia? Presumably doctors would still be free to diagnose and
prescribe within the limits of protocols, but the types and numbers
of cases they handled would be determined by plans submitted for
top management approval by the clinical directorates, while the
standards of their work would be monitored by internal audit that
itself had to win the approval of purchasing authorities.

In fact these are not our predictions. To acknowledge that
management control of health care professionals has been significantly enhanced during the last decade is not at all the same thing as
concluding that such control must continue to grow, sweeping aside
all other forms of power and authority. On the contrary, our
suggestion is that, while some further growth of the management
domain is highly likely, there are also dynamics within this process
which will limit the concentration of control. Furthermore, there is

the point that 'management' itself is certainly not monolithic, and managers are not a single interest group or even ideologically homogeneous. Thus, for example, it is quite conceivable that professionals may acquire management skills without necessarily also embracing a 'managerialist' ideology. To put it in more concrete terms, we may witness the appearance of more and more doctors and nurses who are to some extent management trained but who do not identify themselves with either a management career or the prevailing managerial predilection for economic rationalism.

We see at least seven reasons why the further growth of management control is likely to be constrained. These are, to put them briefly:

● Because professional groups still possess considerable, albeit in some ways diminished, powers to resist managerial control.
● Because NHS hospital managers will become increasingly dependent for finance upon private patients.
● Because the new contractual environment offers some professionals increased opportunity to move away from managerial hierarchies and set up independently.
● Because it will not necessarily be in managers' interests to seek to extend their control into certain areas.
● Because the interests of management are themselves likely to become more fragmented, various and conflictual.
● Because in the longer run, the Government may find that further extension of the powers of managers will not offer them the hoped-for relief from political pressure over the NHS.
● Because (also in the longer run) the empowerment of consumers may begin to create an important new source of legitimacy in NHS politics, challenging management dominance.

It is impossible to attach precise relative weights or probabilities to these seven possible developments, but we are inclined to believe that there is a high *combined* probability that some mixture of them will significantly restrain the further growth of management control. Each of these suggestions deserves further discussion.

## PROFESSIONAL RESISTANCE TO MANAGERIAL CONTROL

Professions are likely to retain considerable autonomy so long as they continue to monopolize their particular skills and control their supply of labour. Thus, for example, managers obviously cannot themselves diagnose patients, and cannot hire any other category of worker (other than a doctor) who can. Doctors therefore continue to control an activity which is highly uncertain (diagnosis is frequently far from straightforward) yet quite fundamental to the flow of work. Managers remain unable to render this activity (and others) predictable, standardized and transparent – and therefore remain largely unable to control it. The use of risky and uncertain activities to create areas of autonomy has long been a theme in organizational studies.[3]

Yet while this is an important argument it is necessary to recognize its limits. There are at least two ways in which management *can* sometimes gain control over initially uncertain and unpredictable activities. First, if the group of workers concerned loses control of the supply of its labour, then managers can easily replace those who attempt to resist the management line, and go on replacing them until they find a group who will conduct the activity in a way that produces results acceptable to top management. Second, technological or scientific advance may make it possible to routinize or automate what was previously an uncertain and highly judgemental task. Both these possibilities have some relevance for the health care professions.

In the case of nursing in particular we have noted how the workforce is likely to be diluted by the creation of health care assistants and by the effective downgrading of existing nursing qualifications when cohorts of the new Project 2000 diplomates begin to appear. Already NHS trusts are able to ignore the recommendations of the Nurses Pay Review Body in the case of nurses employed since their creation. A much more fragmented picture seems likely to emerge in respect to nurses' pay, with a few shortage categories (e.g. theatre nurses in some areas) winning considerable increases but large groups of nurses experiencing strong downward pay pressure from local management. Since nurses' pay accounts for about a quarter of total NHS current spending it constitutes an almost irresistible target for economizers.[4]

In contrast (it might be thought) the medical profession will continue to be able to control the flow of entrants into hospitals and GP surgeries. But this may not be the case. Newspaper reports have recently appeared suggesting that the European Commission has ruled the UK systems of specialist medical training unacceptable, and that it might soon be much easier for continental European specialists (whose training is sometimes shorter than their UK counterparts) to take up NHS posts. Given high levels of medical unemployed in some European countries, an influx would not be unexpected. The Department of Health was said to be planning 'a fundamental overhaul of specialist qualifications and doctors' career structures'.[5]

The reduction of professional judgement to programmable routines or algorithms is the second development which tends to strengthen management's hand. As particular procedures become 'transparent' the professionals who practise them are less able than formerly to argue for diversity of approach and are in principle more susceptible to external performance monitoring. In fact, more and more health care procedures *are* becoming codified in precisely this way. Thus, for example, computer software is now available which will take a doctor step by step through the diagnosis of abdominal pain, drawing on a huge data bank to generate the probabilities of each alternative diagnosis more accurately than most individual clinicians, left to their own devices, could hope to do. Once tools such as this are in existence and known it becomes more hazardous for a doctor to ignore the logical sequence of diagnostic questioning suggested and 'cut corners' to go his or her own way.

What is not clear (at least to non-experts), however, is the extent to which managers will be able and willing to use such developments to their advantage. There are signs that it is usually the profession itself which gains firm control over the new decision aids, which are incorporated within the professional curriculum and declared effectively 'off-limits' to non-professionals.[6] On the other hand, once (say) a recognized professional protocol for the management of a particular condition is published it enables managers to at least question their medical colleagues as to whether the protocol is being fully observed. The scope for individual doctors to 'do it their way' is somewhat lessened, and a new basis for external questioning of particular instances of medical practice is established. One other form of professional resistance must also be mentioned, and that is what one might term the 'counterattack' on burgeoning managerialism. In 1992 the BMA announced (*The Independent*, 7 July 1992: 3) that it was to hold a future conference on rationing, and at its annual conference, its chairperson declared that:

> Clear guidelines must be agreed to bring consistency to medical and surgical priorities throughout the health service.

It seemed clear from this speech that the BMA envisaged *doctors* playing a major role in formulating these priorities. Along with the formation, in 1991, of the British Association of Medical Managers the expression of such sentiments may be taken as significant indicators. They suggest that, if management roles continue to expand, then doctors themselves will seek to occupy many key management positions, and bring their own particular perspectives and interests to bear. How such doctor-managers would behave must remain a fascinating field for future research, but there can surely be no guarantee that they will be as loyal to the messages coming down from the centre as most general managers seem usually to have been. After all, doctor-managers will have, in their medical background, an alternative source of legitimacy (and income) which their purely managerial counterparts do not.

## HOSPITAL DEPENDENCE UPON PRIVATE PATIENTS

In an environment of competition between provider units for cash-limited resources, small changes in patient flows are financially important because of a hospital's typically high level of fixed and semi-fixed costs. Of double importance, therefore, is revenue from treating private patients in NHS paybeds: not only a welcome addition to funds, but from outside the cash limit. But it is difficult for a hospital directly to attract private patients (though perceived poor facilities may repel them!) and in practice it must rely on doctors to fill paybeds rather than sending private cases to the local private hospitals. Thus, to some extent, managers are reciprocally dependent on doctors.

It is true, of course, that Trust hospitals may change consultants' conditions of service so as to forbid their taking private cases elsewhere, but that cannot of itself maximize private cases brought to NHS hospitals. Moreover, the private health care industry may well respond to NHS competition by encouraging the whole-time practice of private medicine within private hospitals, ensuring that it obtains business by offering preferential terms to insured patients. In summary, therefore, those doctors who practise in specialties where substantial private work is available will have resources with which to bargain against NHS managers.[7]

If, at some point in the future, NHS Trusts were to be sold in order to help sustain the Government's income from privatization proceeds (which, on current forecasts, peak in 1992–93: see Chapter 2), buy-outs of provider institutions by joint groups of managers and doctors would be a strong possibility. If this were to occur, it would create an obvious realignment of the currently somewhat opposed interests of the two groups.

## ESCAPE FROM THE HIERARCHY: THE GROWTH OF INDEPENDENT PROFESSIONAL GROUPINGS

Straightforward (or subtle) resistance to managerial hierarchies is not, however, the only strategy open to health care professionals seeking to preserve their autonomy. Another option would be to move out with the main organizational structures and then operate as an independent partnership or firm, hiring services back to the main purchasing or providing agencies. In a sense this is what GPs – notoriously *the* least regimented branch of the medical profession – have done since 1948. The prospect now is that the model may be copied much more widely. Groups of office-based consultants could hire themselves out to fundholding GPs and secondary providers on negotiated terms. It is not impossible that other professional groups could follow – physiotherapists and occupational therapists, for example. Nursing agencies are already a feature of the scene, and could multiply and adopt new forms. Indeed, such developments would be very much within the spirit of the new 'contract culture'. Parallel trends can be identified in other public services: the contracting out of professional services in local authorities and in the post 'Next Steps' civil service; the rapid increase in the use of part-time contracted academic staff in institutions of higher education.[8] Perhaps the most obvious example of all is the US health care system, where office-based doctors with practising rights in a variety of local hospitals are the norm.

This is not at all to imply that increasing contracting out of core professional services will always and without exception represent a gain in professional autonomy and an escape from managerialist controls. The picture is likely to be much more mixed. For some professional groups the nominal status of independent local provider will bring little autonomy. If there is a dominant local purchaser and plenty of competing professional groups exist the purchaser may be able to drive a hard bargain and insist on strict terms and controls. But there will surely be many instances where these conditions do not hold. Much demand for health care is supplier-induced, so that high status groups of consultants offering rare specialist skills may be able to exploit their market niche and, to a substantial degree, choose their own location and working hours. In short, a much more openly variegated picture than we have hitherto been accustomed to is likely to emerge. Those professional groups with market advantages will be able to 'moor offshore' of the main NHS providers and hire themselves back at favourable rates. Those groups without such advantages may find themselves contracted out against their will, and subject to tightly-drawn terms and conditions. These possibilities of professionals opting out of the hierarchy would be much enhanced if there were to occur a substantial expansion of the private health care market in the UK, whether as a result of public disillusionment with the NHS (were such to occur) or of Government policy changes in relation to tax relief on health insurance subscriptions.

## HOW FAR WILL MANAGERS WANT TO GO?

A fourth limitation to the further extension of managerial control is likely to be the perceived self interest of the managers themselves. Will they *want* total control? The answer is almost certainly no.

As we noted in Chapter 1, there is a sense in which professional autonomy is in the interest of government. Whilst the forces described in Chapter 2 point towards an unavoidable intensification of the rationing of health care services, and while managers may be the Government's chosen instrument for achieving control of the process, most managers are understandably reluctant to take direct responsibility for rationing decisions themselves. Such decisions are invariably controversial, sometimes intensely so, and managers are not spectacularly more willing than politicians to take public and personal responsibility for unpopular choices. A measure of clinical autonomy is therefore protective of managers, as well as of politicians. At the grass roots level managers have shown no enthusiasm for taking over decisions about offering or not offering individuals treatment. By and large managers remain content to uphold the convenient fiction that these decisions are purely medical/scientific (despite the fact that research indicates that social judgements are often intricately interwoven with medical ones, e.g. in decisions whether to offer dialysis to the elderly).

At a more aggregated level, however, managers in purchasing authorities do seem to have become more willing to set explicit priorities. These have included tightly limiting, or in some cases no longer purchasing certain treatments. Typically these have been treatments regarded as 'cosmetic' and/or 'ineffective'. Even here, however, managers have been careful to involve doctors in the decisions and to cloak them, as far as possible, with clinical legitimacy (though again, 'effectiveness' is ultimately a social and political rather than a medical judgement). It often seems that managers' ideal position would be one in which they are able to determine the 'formulae' or broad priorities for rationing, but continue to avoid the stress which accompanies taking responsibility for the actual application of such guidelines to the mass of individual cases. Clearly there are persuasive arguments for managers performing exactly such a role. In practice, however, it may prove a state of grace which is very hard to attain. Not only may the established priorities be overturned by political interventions (as when a minister does not like the headlined consequences of the application of a particular priority) but the managers themselves may be increasingly challenged by the doctor-managers mentioned above. Given the history and habits of the NHS it is not at all unlikely that in so far as explicit rationing rules *are* formulated, this will be done at a high level, with much to-ing and fro-ing between the DoH, the BMA and the royal colleges.

Foreseeing this, it is likely that many managers will fudge the establishment of clear priorities in the first place. Without explicit – and durable – political backing the taking of such responsibility would leave the managers concerned in an exposed position. Thus even the formulation of general guidelines is likely to be approached with great caution, and pursued only where a reasonable consensus can be manufactured with the relevant medical and political interests.


## THE FRAGMENTATION OF 'MANAGEMENT'

A further limit to the expansion of managerial power and authority is set by the fact that 'management' itself is not a single, monolithic interest. Indeed, it may well be that accelerating decentralization and competition within a provider market (to the extent that these come about) will lead to greater fragmentation of management than the NHS was accustomed to during the later 1980s and early 1990s.

The main cleavages within 'management' are already visible. There is an obvious one between purchaser management and provider management – potentially a deeper cleavage than the old divides between regions and districts or districts and units. There is another between the managements of competing provider institutions, each striving to increase its own market share. And there is a third between top management and middle management. This divide is not unique to the NHS, and is beginning to emerge as a focus for considerable theoretical interest among academics.[9] Rationally self-interested top management is less concerned with maximizing service provision (and therefore spending) than with politically-determined status, with *control* of the overall system and with maintaining the (often quite small) core budget which supports their own top level operations. Middle management, however, is necessarily much more closely involved with the day-to-day provision of services and therefore with the programme budget which finances those services. Thus it may be in the interests of top managers to please ministers and enhance their control and status by making sweeping reorganizations and enthusiastically implementing further efficiency drives. The effects of such activities – indeed, their very point from a ministerial point of view – may be programme budget reductions. Such changes, while they demonstrate the power of top managers (who take care to preserve their own core budgets), often spell uncomfortable career changes for middle management, if not actual redundancy. Indeed, 'squeezing out' middle management has become a kind of virility symbol in the iconography of top private sector management in the 1990s, just as 'taking on the unions' did during the preceding decade.[10]

Within the specific context of the NHS mid-rank career administrators currently have good reason to be anxious, since their roles are subject to increasing competition from professionals-turned-managers, especially clinical directors and nurse-managers. The enhanced powers of top management may, for reasons given above, make the lives of middle managers even more precarious. Certainly an analysis based solely on a simple bipolar division between 'managers' and 'professionals' would be too crude to take us very far. A more convincing picture of the future would include various groups *within* management and other groups *within* each major

profession manoeuvring for advantage across the new organizational terrain populated by different kinds of purchasers and
providers. During these manoeuvres a variety of alliances (e.g.
between local middle managers and local consultants versus top
management) are likely to come into being, with the pattern still
further complicated by the above-mentioned possibility that some
professionals may recompose themselves as independent providers,
at arms length even from the main provider units.

## STRENGTHENING MANAGEMENT'S HAND MAY NO LONGER SEEM SO ADVANTAGEOUS TO GOVERNMENT

The rise of management relative to the professions since the early
1980s has been driven more by the needs of central government
than by any other single factor. In the NHS general managers have
been, above all else, the implementers of the policies handed down
by the Department of Health and its Scottish, Welsh and Northern
Irish counterparts. So long as managers remain useful in this respect
so long may they reasonably expect their general status to continue
to advance. But what if, after a few years, the current portfolio of
policies (purchaser/provider split, etc.) did not appear to be
contributing to the solution of the strategic political and policy
problems discussed in Chapter 2?

In fact we do not have to wait that long to see how careless
ministers can be with managers' sensitivities. All politicians, but
particularly those of the 'New Right' enjoy criticizing 'bureaucracy'.
In 1991 the then Secretary of State for Health was to be heard
publicly praising GP fundholding because it was better than giving
money to 'bureaucrats' in the districts and regions. This was but the
latest of a long line of speeches in which ministers had emphasized
the need to cut back on 'bureaucracy' in favour of the doctors and
nurses at the 'sharp end' – the popularity of this theme not waning in
the face of evidence that NHS administrative costs were actually
startlingly *low* compared with those of the more market-oriented
US system. Although the present Secretary of State has reaffirmed
political support for the DHA purchasing function, there can be no
guarantee that this support will endure.[11]

Ministers themselves would no doubt draw (as they have in the
past) a strong distinction between 'needless bureaucracy' and

'energetic management serving the patient'. But there are several difficulties with this formulation. First, the distinction between the two may be anything but clear on the ground – often more a matter of vantage point than systematic evidence. Second, ministers have to be wary of the survey evidence which indicates that in general the public trusts doctors and nurses far more than either managers/ administrators or themselves.[12] Third, critics of the 1989 White Paper have had some success in establishing in the public mind the idea that the provider market reforms have been accompanied by a great proliferation of managers and accountants. Whether this is correct or not it has helped tie management's fortunes closely to the perceived success (or failure) of the reforms. If the NHS is still seen as 'in crisis' in the mid-1990s it is far from clear that ministers would stand by management if there were to be a 1987–88-style wave of media and public criticism. These comments are, of course, extremely speculative. They are principally intended to underline the basic point that the particular political powers which have fostered the growth to prominence of the management function are ultimately fickle ones. It would be an unwarrantedly optimistic manager who suggested that the kind of ministerial support for managers evinced since the 1989 White Paper will continue indefinitely or irrespective of wider circumstances.

## CONSUMER EMPOWERMENT?

The final development which could constrain the further growth of management dominance is the possible emergence of a real user voice in a service which was until recently ingrained with paternalism. As we have already discussed 'consumerism' in Chapter 5 and elsewhere just a few possibilities for the future will be drawn out here.

It will be clear from our earlier analysis that we do not envisage the sudden transformation of the NHS into an organization driven by expressed user needs or measured against standards or criteria the formulation of which has been largely shaped by the consumer's voice. Developments thus far seems more often to take the form of numerous and various local surveys of user opinion, the data from which is then employed by management as an ancillary source of legitimacy to support changes to traditional practices and arrangements. Consumer 'choice' in the new system may well have been somewhat enlarged (it was extremely circumscribed previously) but in total remains modest. On the whole the patient still follows the money (now in the form of block or cost-and-volume contracts) rather than vice versa.

For these reasons we do not see consumers' opinions and priorities soon becoming a major constraint on management. But neither do we see them as totally insignificant. The wider availability of information about user preferences offers a resource to professionals as well as managers. Also, within the management hierarchy, it is likely to provide ammunition to middle- and coal-face management in their struggle to convince top management that they need resources. Already these processes are visible across a number of public services, e.g. in higher education where student opinion gathered in surveys is being deployed by lecturers and others to argue for better libraries, more student accommodation, no further increases in seminar group sizes, and so on. They represent the modest intrusion of a third form of legitimacy into *internal* debates about public services (the first two being professional authority and political authority as transmitted downwards through the management hierarchy).

It remains impossible to be sure how, or how far, this third form of legitimacy will be deployed. At present it appears to function principally as a resource to groups *other* than the users themselves – to managers, doctors, nurses, etc. Promoting direct use by users would appear to require, *inter alia*, reinforcement of users' formal representative mechanisms – by strengthening Community Health Councils or creating some new body. This would be contrary to the government's current beliefs about the relative usefulness of 'voice' and 'choice', and has not appeared high on ministers' agendas for a decade or more. If we assume that direct collective representation of users' views is *not* noticeably enhanced in the near future then the question becomes one of which group or groups will succeed in wielding consumer satisfaction data to the greatest advantage. The answer could easily vary from one locality to another, depending on a variety of contingencies. Certainly it is by no means a foregone conclusion that top management, though they may have been instrumental in launching the wave of consumer surveys, will be able to retain control of the 'product'.

## CONCLUDING REMARKS

In this final chapter we have attempted to provide glimpses of some possible futures for work and organization in the NHS. Taken together they suggest a kind of 'elastic net' restraining the indefinite extension of the management domain and the indefinite curtailment of professional autonomy. The first five chapters show that the management domain *has* grown rapidly in the recent past. This sixth chapter argues that, while some further growth is likely, there are limits and countervailing tendencies.

The image of an elastic net is appropriate in that it has no one fixed form, but it does have certain overall tolerances. The glimpses of possible futures we have described (more fragmented management, some growth of independent groups of professionals, a struggle over the meaning of user data, etc.) do not add up to a single portrait of 'how it will be'. Rather we suggest that the future politics of the NHS will very probably revolve around certain basic dilemmas which are anything but new. These include the political salience of the NHS, the unavoidability of rationing, the sensitivity (and frequent unpopularity) of specific rationing decisions, the continuing uncertainty of basic medical procedures such as diagnosis and choice of individual therapy, the high rate of change of health care technologies and the ability of highly-trained, extremely intelligent professionals to evade, deflect or delay attempts to standardize or externally monitor their activities.

The provider market may be new but many of the problems it will have to embrace are thus venerable ones. The evolution and re-design of the relationships between different units and different groups of staff are already giving birth to genuine novelties and new departures. Yet these new relationships have somehow still to stretch round the old problems. It is in the middle of a period of intense bending, stretching and re-positioning that we are obliged to leave you.

# NOTES

## 1 Professionals and managers

1 On the character of professionalism, see Johnson (1972) and Esland (1980). Etzioni (1969) examines the 'semi-professions'. For critical histories of the UK health professions, see Parry and Parry (1976) on medicine; Abel-Smith (1961) on nursing; and Larkin (1983) on opticians, radiographers, physiotherapists and chiropodists.
2 On the 'new nursing', see Salvage (1992).
3 See Pollitt (1993).
4 See, for example, Niskanen (1973).
5 For a broad overview of quality concepts and techniques see Centre for the Evaluation of Public Policy and Practice (1992a).
6 On performance indicators, see Audit Commission (1991). On competition, see H.M. Treasury (1991).

## 2 Finance for health care: supply, demand and rationing

1 For a basic introduction to theory in the social sciences, see Pollitt (1991). For its application to the organization and management of the NHS, see Harrison, Hunter and Pollitt (1990, Chapter 1).
2 The 'age of discontinuity' quotation is from Drucker (1982). For Marxist theories about the future of the Welfare State, see Offe (1984) and O'Connor (1973). For a more general analysis of relevant aspects of the future, see Handy (1985, 1989). For the relationship between 'hard' and 'soft' variables, see Vickers (1965) and Young (1977).
3 Gross *National* Product, sometimes used in international expenditure comparisons, adds to GDP 'net property income from abroad' to UK residents. In the specific case of the UK there is little absolute difference

between GDP and GNP. (It is worth noting that GDP/GNP are not uncontested as ways of valuing a country's economic activity. They are highly materialistic and takes no account of non-remunerated activity such as housework or DIY.) Many factors are, of course, involved in the determination of GDP. They include microeconomic factors (such as industrial efficiency) as well as macroeconomic ones such as inflation. For accessible accounts, see Donaldson and Farquhar (1988) and Levacic (1987).

4 For details of the 'cash limit' system of public expenditure control introduced in the UK in the 1970s, see Henley *et al.* (1986), and Likierman (1988). The reader will find helpful information in Thain and Wright (1991) and Flynn (1990).

5 The other end, as it were, of the increasing proportion of elderly persons in the UK is the reducing proportion (and, as it happens, absolute number) of younger age groups. (See Table 2.2.) This has provided a partial rationale for the process of deskilling the professions which we touch upon in Chapter 3.

6 The calculations for the costs of importing US levels of technology utilisation to the UK are taken from Aaron and Schwartz (1984, Table 5.1). It is important to remember that the whole exercise assumes the desirability of such a process, which is far from self-evident.

As distinct from technical developments, for the financial year 1986/87 the DHSS estimated that (Robinson and Judge 1987):

> The level of spending required to improve services will depend on decisions as to specific policy objectives over the period. In the current year these are estimated at some half of one per cent.

The degree of consensus about this second half per cent is less clear, and we have, therefore omitted it from our calculations for Figure 2.5. For an entertaining account of how medical professionals by-pass managers in the introduction of new technology, see Council for Science and Society (1982).

7 Our calculations in respect of the 'efficiency trap' all use English figures. For an illustrated discussion of the concept, see Green and Harrison (1989). The careful reader will have noted the quotes around the phrase 'treating more patients' in the main text. Even with the Körner definition of 'finished consultant episodes' it is far from clear how many readmissions are contained within these figures. If Oxford Region is typical of the remainder of the country, re-admission rates have increased substantially: see Henderson *et al.* (1989). (In addition to efficiency savings, a small amount of money, £10 million in 1988–89, is raised by NHS income generation schemes, such as renting hospital space to shops.)

8 The National Association of Health Authorities and Trusts commissions annual polls of public opinion concerning the NHS. For

comparisons between different sectors of the welfare state see Taylor-Gooby (1985, 1987). For a selection of opinion poll findings about health professionals, see Harrison (1988).

9 On approaches to rationing, see Boyd (1979), Smith (1992), Heginbotham (1992), Stewart (1990) and Klein (1992).

10 On alternative possible approaches to financing the NHS, see Institute of Health Services Management (1988).

Between 1979 and 1986 UK *public* expenditure on health care grew from 4.7 per cent of GDP to 5.3 per cent, whilst private expenditure grew from 0.5 per cent to 0.8 per cent (Laing 1988).

11 For a questioning approach to the genuineness of 'cost-improvements' in the NHS, see National Audit Office (1986).

12 The NHS Pay and Prices Index represents price changes in the 'basket of goods' that a hospital or health services institutions might purchase; it is thus analogous to the Retail Prices Index for a household. In practice, the NHS index increases more rapidly than either retail prices or the other inflation measure, the GDP deflator, frequently quoted by official sources.

## 3 Challenging the professionals

1 On the parameters of 'clinical freedom', see Schulz and Harrison (1986) and Tolliday (1978). For a selection of UK government statements on the topic, see Harrison (1988), Chapter 2. The NHS as the aggregate of individual clinical decisions is well demonstrated by Haywood and Alaszewski (1980), Chapter 5. For a more general statement of the argument, see Lipsky (1980). For an analysis of occupational control in health 'manpower' planning, see Harrison (1981) and Harrison, Hunter and Pollitt (1990), Chapter 4. Watkin (1975) reprints extracts from a number of relevant reports. Sir Lancelot Spratt stalks the pages of Dr Richard Gordon's *Doctor in the House* (memorably played by James Robertson Justice in the film version) and its sequelae.

2 For a more extensive summary of research findings on pre-Griffiths NHS management, together with fully-referenced sources, see Harrison (1988), Chapter 3. For an analysis of the relationship between the research findings and the Griffiths diagnosis, see Harrison (1988), Chapter 4.

3 For an account of the formalities and operation of NHS consensus, see Harrison (1982).

4 For a discussion of accountability in the context of public services, see Day and Klein (1987).

5 For an analysis of team consensus decision-making in the NHS, see S. Harrison (1982, 1984).

6 For more detailed accounts of the Griffiths recommendations, see Harrison (1988) and Levitt and Wall (1992).

7 The sources for these research findings, together with a more detailed summary, may be found in Harrison, Hunter, Marnoch and Pollitt (1992).

8 For an elaborate demonstration of the impossibility of managerial understanding of the whole of an organization's operations, see Dunsire (1978).

9 The DHSS performance indicators were originally developed in isolation from pre-existing academic work along the same lines, though eventually integrated with it: see Yates (1983).

10 For critiques of the original performance indicators, see Pollitt (1985a,b), Mullen (1985) and Brotherton (1985) for the basis of the notion of medically preventable death, see Charlton *et al*. (1983).

11 See Carter *et al*. (1992: 169). This book contains much useful discussion of the 'politics of information'.

12 The DHSS was split into separate Departments of Health (DoH), and Social Security, in 1988.

13 Research evidence about the use of performance indicators and other forms of management information may be found in Jenkins *et al*. (1987) and Pollitt *et al*. (1988). Some exceptions to the general trend indicated by these studies may be found in Day (1989).

14 For general assessments of industrial relations in the NHS up to the mid-1980s see Barnard and Harrison (1986) and Mailly *et al*. (1989). The most up-to-date account is Seifert (1992).

15 For additional details of the 1982 dispute, see Mailly *et al*. (1989).

16 For details of the Review Body and other aspects of the formalities of NHS industrial relations at national level, see Harrison (1989). The occupations other than nursing which are covered by the Review Body are physiotherapy, radiography, occupational therapy, orthoptics, chiropody and dietetics.

17 For a range of contemporary views about the merits of local flexibility in pay determination, see the special Centre Eight issue of *Health and Social Service Journal*, 3 October 1985.

18 For a discussion of industrial relations in the early NHS Trusts, see Hodges (1991).

19 For a critical discussion of nursing workload measures, see Jenkins-Clarke and Carr-Hill (1991). Related quality assurance systems are well-described in Sale (1990).

20 See National Audit Office (1985).

21 Individual 'job plans' for hospital consultants were introduced after 1989 (Starkey 1992). Rather than controlling staff numbers, these were aimed at ensuring that doctors fulfilled their contractual hours.

22 For an account of the saga of the consultant/junior ratio, see Harrison, Hunter and Pollitt (1990).

23 For an account of the relationships between medicine and some of the paramedical professions see Larkin (1983). For a discussion of the claim

that medical knowledge 'overarches' that of other health professions, see Tolliday (1978).

24 See the Medicinal Products (Prescribing by Nurses) Act 1992.

25 The NVQ system, despite widespread acceptance, has been criticized by professions who fear its eventual effect on their own occupational control as higher-level qualifications begin to be accredited: see *Industrial Relations Review and Report*, No. 394, 1989.

26 Salvage (1992) and McKee and Lessof (1992).

## 4 Incorporating the professionals

1 This form of corporatism is sometimes termed 'liberal corporatism' to distinguish it from its employment as a tactic of totalitarian regimes. For a review, see Grant (1985), Chapters 1 and 2. For a case study which casts doubt on the ability of the medical profession to control its rank and file, see Harrison, Hunter and Pollitt (1990), Chapter 4. For the general application of corporatist theory to the NHS and other sectors of the welfare state, see Cawson (1982) and M.L. Harrison (1984).

2 For a series of studies of 'meso-corporatism' below national level, see Cawson (1985). Rhodes (1986) reached the conclusion that corporatism was merely a tactic in central government financial relationships with local government.

3 Unlike Ham and Hunter (1988: 7) and Hunter (1992: 558) we do not take the view that such approaches as medical audit are *necessarily* the 'minimal' strategy for managing doctors; they may be the proverbial 'thin end of the wedge'.

4 For a general discussion of RM in the NHS, see Perrin (1988), Pinch *et al.* (1989) and Symes (1992).

5 For an accessible account of DRGs in the UK, see Bardsley *et al.* (1987). For updates, see the periodic *Diagnosis Related Groups Newsletter*. For a comprehensive treatment of the conceptual and technical bases of casemix, see Hornbrook (1982).

6 For more details of early work with clinical budgets, see Wickings *et al.* (1983) and Wickings (1983).

7 Arthur Young (1986); Pollitt *et al.* (1988).

8 The DHSS's review of MB may be found in DHSS (1986).

9 Our evidence of the impact of RM is largely drawn from Pollitt *et al.* (1988), Pinch *et al.* (1989), Scrivens (1988), Flynn (1988) and, most importantly, from the formal evaluation of the pilot sites, Packwood *et al.* (1991).

10 For medical involvement in the NHS, see Harrison (1988), Chapter 2. The three categories are drawn from Perey (1984).

11 For discussion of doctors as career managers, see Hunter (1992), Leathard (1990), Stewart *et al.* (1987) and Harrison (1988). As Schulz and Johnson (1990: 3) note, salaried medically qualified directors are

common in American hospitals. In some countries, such a qualification is the norm for health service management.

12 There has sometimes been a degree of shared hierarchy within the health professions, for instance between physiotherapy and occupational therapy. In some cases, there was an ambiguous relationship between doctors in the diagnostic specialties and the professional heads of radiography and medical laboratory sciences.

13 Despite being implemented in the 1970s, it was not until 1984 that the Johns Hopkins model was widely publicized, through an article in the *New England Journal of Medicine* (Heyssel *et al*. 1984). It is one of the ironies of the English/American 'common' language, that 'administration' in the latter case does not carry the pejorative (low-status, routine, bureaucratic) connotations found (indeed, since Griffiths, actively promoted) in the UK.

14 For reviews of the clinical directorate model, see Packwood *et al*. (1992), Fitzgerald (1991a,b) and Disken *et al*. (1990); see also Ham and Hunter (1988: 22).

15 The internal re-organization into 'clinical directorates' (or whatever) pose a considerable threat to the traditional role of the bureaucratic middle manager. First, like any form of decentralization, it removes the filtering and coordination function from these middle levels. Second, these changes remove traditional career/promotion opportunities within a clearly defined hierarchy.

16 See Watkin (1978), Chapter 5.

17 Since the mid-1980s the volume of publications on quality in health care services has expanded very rapidly. It is doubly hard to keep track of because much of it is in the form of locally issued and sometimes ephemeral pamphlets, handbooks, etc. or even rather expensive videos (at the time of writing the NHS Management Executive/NAHAT video on quality cost more than £100). Nevertheless there are cheaper, more durable and more widely-available sources. As general background we would recommend Pfeffer and Coote (1991) as a stimulating introduction to the fashion for quality and the battle over meanings. In the private sector, and to a lesser extent in the public, British Standard BS5750 (defining quality system requirements) has been influential. This is concisely described in the DTI booklet *BS5750/ISO 9000: 1987: A Positive Contribution to Better Business* (1989). In 1992, a Leicester GP surgery became the first general practice to receive the British Standards Institute 'kitemark', signifying that it had satisfied BS5750.

18 More specific treatments of the NHS include the National Audit Office (1988) which gives an overall picture immediately prior to the *Working for Patients* White Paper.

19 On practice variations, see Anderson and Mooney (1990). The Edinburgh experience is reported in Gruer *et al*. (1986) and many subsequent publications. GP experience is reported in Russell *et al*.

(1992). Other examples are given in Ham and Hunter (1988: 11–13). For a review of approaches to medical audit, see Hopkins (1991).

20 For an important study of clinical consensus, see Lomas (1991).

21 The original CEPOD report is Buck *et al.* (1987); the first national CEPOD is Royal College of Surgeons (1990).

22 Medical audit has spawned a number of publications, particularly by the royal colleges. A good early example was the Royal College of Physicians (1989). A concise review of the different views of medical audit which were in play during the early 1990s was Packwood (1991). Many health authorities produced documents of their own, one of the most thoughtful being Frater and Spiby (1990) for the North West Thames Regional Health Authority.

23 Despite some work by Stocking (1992) and Russell *et al.* (1992), the relationship between audit and behaviour change is markedly under-researched in comparison to such matters as audit processes and information systems.

24 The government has just recently announced a new set of six publicly available performance indicators for hospitals. These are all process measures, such as waiting times, though there are plans for later extension 'to include clinical indicators such as re-admission rates after a treatment goes wrong'. See *The Times*, 24 February 1993, 1–2.

25 The literature on nursing quality is vast. Much of it is North American, but two useful starting places among the more specifically British texts are Sale (1990) and the Royal College of Nursing (1989). The survey of quality initiatives referred to is Dalley and Carr-Hill (1991).

26 See Centre for the Evaluation of Public Policy and Practice (1991, 1992b).

## 5 Changing the environment

1 For an extensive discussion of the theoretical relationship of an organiz-ation to its environment, see Pfeffer and Salancik (1978). For details of staffing changes 1931–91, see Brindle (1993).

2 Alternative terms for 'purchasing' are 'commissioning', 'acquiring' and 'enabling'.

3 See Enthoven (1985a,b). For his US related policy prescriptions, see especially Enthoven (1978).

4 Working for Patients (Department of Health 1989) was the product of a prime ministerial review of the NHS. Originally established in response to a perceived funding crisis, the review succeeded in sidestepping the funding issue and concentrating on structural reform. For one account, see Griggs (1991). Note that Figure 5.2, and subsequent textual remarks about NHS organization, employ English terminology. The same gen-eral arrangements, with differences of detail and of terminology, apply in Scotland and Wales: see Levitt and Wall (1992).

5 Despite the existence of deliberately alternative terms (e.g. 'service agreements'), the term 'contract' (like 'poll tax') has stuck.

6 We discussed some of the consequences of the additional freedoms granted to NHS Trusts in Chapter 3; for details of Trust constitution, etc. see Levitt and Wall (1992).

7 For a basic account of the HMO principle, see Culyer *et al*. (1988). For reviews of US experience with this form of organization, see Hornbrook and Berki (1985), Weiner and Ferriss (1990), Feldman *et al*. (1990) and Ware *et al*. (1986).

8 For details of the GP fundholding scheme, see Glennerster *et al*. (1992).

9 For a compelling attempt at theorizing the state of affairs represented by this cliché, see Kingdon (1984).

10 For outlines of comparable developments in some other European countries, see Saltman and von Otter (1987, 1989, 1990, 1992), World Health Organization (1989) and Saltman *et al*. (1990).

11 For an analysis of quasi-markets in the welfare state generally, see LeGrand (1990).

12 The general basis of the belief that bureaucrats are 'empire builders' may be found in Niskanen (1971). For a comprehensive critique of this and associated ideas, see Dunleavy (1991).

13 In the early period of operation of the purchaser/provider split, this problem has been partially circumvented by the use of 'block contracts', which do not entail detailed specification of cases or prices. But since this is widely held to work against the interests of provider institutions (who thereby do *not* receive more money for more patients) it is likely that the future will see greater use on 'cost and volume' contracts which do specify numbers and types of case.

14 See, for instance, *Yorkshire Post*, 22 April 1992, p. 9.

15 See Jones (1992).

16 Other new forms of leverage include the requirement that consultants cannot qualify for distinction awards unless they demonstrate 'commitment to the management and development of the service' (Department of Health 1989: 44).

17 See, for example, Limb (1992).

18 Capitation fees are the element of a GP's income related to list size: a fixed annual fee (which varies with the patient's age) irrespective of work actually performed for the patient.

19 Figures showing public satisfaction with GPs are published annually by the National Association of Health Authorities and Trusts. A typical figure is 90 per cent satisfied.

20 See Appleby *et al*. (1992: 9–10).

21 See, for instance, Tomlin (1992), Ham and Heginbotham (1992). On 'locality purchasing', see Ham (1992).

22 Day and Klein (1991) calculated that extension of fundholding to all English GPs, but without extending the items purchased by the funds,

would cost £3.2 billion in 1991 prices. This is more than 13 per cent of the total cost of the NHS: GP prescribing accounts for a further 11 per cent. To these items must be added the costs of capitation fees and other payments to GPs, as well as the extension of liability of GP fundholders to pay for community nursing from 1993.

23 At least one DHA and Family Health Service Authority (FHSA) share a chief executive. Moreover, the merger of DHAs is likely to produce a *de facto* co-terminosity with FHSAs.

24 See Williamson (1992).

25 See O'Sullivan (1992).

## 6 The future of managerial and professional work in the NHS

1 Readers may recognize this as the 'person culture' elaborated by Charles Handy in his widely-used book, *Understanding Organisations*. For a discussion of cultural change in the NHS see Harrison *et al*. (1992).

2 See, for instance, Long and Sheldon (1992).

3 For example, Crozier (1964).

4 Buchan (1992).

5 For discussion of European qualifications, see Jones (1992). On medical unemployment, see Viefhues (1988).

6 On abdominal pain, see de Dombal *et al*. (1972). The systematization of professional decision-making is a fairly technical area, difficult for the layperson to comprehend. The flavour of it may be tasted in Dowie and Elstein (1988). A lively introduction to the whole field is the Open University course *D321: Professional Judgement*.

7 On the basics of costing, see Perrin (1988). For an example of an NHS Trust restricting consultants' private practice, see Tomlin (1993). The for-profit private health insurance industry in the UK has begun both competitive marketing and is planning cost controls: see, for instance, *The Guardian*, 26 February 1992, p. 2 and Laing (1992).

8 See, for example, H.M. Treasury (1991: 12–13), *The Guardian*, 1 June 1992, p. 1, and *Personal Management Plus*, December 1992, p. 1.

9 See, for example, Dunleavy, P. (1989).

10 See, for example, Kanter (1990). RHAs are making savage cuts in their staffing complements.

11 Davies (1992). See also *The Times*, 24 February 1993, pp. 1–2.

12 Harrison (1988).

# REFERENCES

Aaron, H.J. and Schwartz, W.B. (1984) *The Painful Prescription: Rationing Hospital Care*. Brookings Institution, Washington DC.

Abel-Smith, B. (1961) *A History of the Nursing Profession*. Heinemann, London.

Anderson, T.F. and Mooney, G. (1990) *The Challenge of Medical Practice Variations*. Macmillan, Basingstoke.

Appleby, J., Little, V., Ranadé, W. *et al.* (1992) *Implementing the Reforms: a Second National Survey of District General Managers*. National Association of Health Authorities and Trusts, Birmingham.

Audit Commission (1991) *Citizen's Charter Performance Indicators*. Audit Commission, London.

Bardsley, M., Coles, J. and Jenkins, L. (eds) (1987) *DRGs and Health Care: The Management of Case Mix*. King's Fund, London.

Barnard, K. and Harrison, S. (1986) 'Labour relations in health services management', *Social Science and Medicine*, 22(11): 1213–28.

Boyd, K.M. (ed.) (1979) *The Ethics of Resource Allocation in Health Care*. University of Edinburgh Press, Edinburgh.

Brindle, D. (1993) 'Market is strangling NHS with red tape, MP claims', *The Guardian*, 7 January, p. 5.

Brotherton, P.G. (1985) 'How to make statistics count', *Hospital and Health Services Review*, 81(5): 226–9.

Buchan, J. (1992) *Prospects for Nurses' Pay: 'Flexibility or Fragmentation?'*. King's Fund Institute, London.

Buck, N., Devlin, B. and Lunn, J.N. (1987) *Report of a Confidential Enquiry into Perioperative Deaths*. Nuffield Provincial Hospitals Trust, London.

Carter, N., Klein, R.E. and Day, P. (1992) *How Organisations Measure Success: The Use of Performance Indicators in Government*. Routledge, London.

Cawson, A. (1982) *Corporatism and Welfare: Social Policy and State Intervention in Britain.* Heinemann Education Books, London.

Cawson, A. (1985) 'Varieties of corporatism: the importance of the meso-level of interest intermediation'. In Cawson, A. (ed.) *Organisational Interests and the State: Studies in Meso-Corporatism,* Sage, London.

Centre for the Evaluation of Public Policy and Practice (1991) *Evaluation of Total Quality Management Projects in the National Health Service: First Interim Report to Department of Health.* Brunel University, Uxbridge.

Centre for the Evaluation of Public Policy and Practice (1992a) *Considering Quality: An Analytical Guide to the Literature on Quality and Standards in the Public Services.* Brunel University, Uxbridge.

Centre for the Evaluation of Public Policy and Practice (1992b) *Evaluation of Total Quality Management Projects in the National Health Service: Second Interim Report to the Department of Health.* Brunel University, Uxbridge.

Charlton, J.R.H., Silver, R., Hartley, R.M. and Holland, W.W. (1983) 'Geographical variations in mortality from conditions amenable to medical intervention in England and Wales', *The Lancet,* 25 March.

Coles, J. (1986) 'The myths and realities of DRGs in the NHS', *Hospital and Health Services Review,* 82(1): 28–31.

Committee of Public Accounts, Seventh Report (1981) *Session 1980–81: Financial Control and Accountability in the National Health Service.* House of Commons/HMSO, London.

Council for Science and Society (1982) *Expensive Medical Techniques.* CSS, London.

Crozier, M. (1964) *The Bureaucratic Phenomenon.* University of Chicago Press, Chicago.

Culyer, A.J., Donaldson, C. and Gerard, K. (1988) *Alternatives for Funding Health Services in the UK.* Institute of Health Services Management, London.

Dalley, G. and Carr-Hill, R. (1991) *Pathways to quality: A Study of Quality Management Initiatives in the NHS.* University of York Centre for Health Economics, York.

Davies, P. (1992) 'Musical chairs to the election tune', *Health Service Journal,* 12 March, p. 8.

Day, C. (1989) *Taking Action with Indicators.* HMSO, London.

Day, P. and Klein, R.E. (1991) *Political Theory and Policy Practice: The Case of General Practice 1911–1991,* Paper presented at the Political Studies Association Conference, Lancaster, 15–17 April.

Day, P. and Klein, R.E. (1987) *Accountabilities: Five Public Services.* Tavistock, London.

De Dombal, F.T., Leaper, D.J., Staniland, J.R. *et al.* (1972) 'Computer-aided diagnosis of acute abdominal pain', *British Medical Journal,* (2): 9–13.

Department of Health and Social Security (1986), *Health Services Management: Resource Management (Management Budgeting) in Health Authorities*, Circular HN(86)34.

Department of Health, Welsh Office, Scottish Home and Health Department and Northern Ireland Office (1989) *Working for Patients*, Cm. 555. HMSO, London.

DHSS and Welsh Office (1979) *Patients First: Consultative Document on Structure and Management of the NHS in England and Wales*. HMSO, London.

Disken, S., Dixon, M., Halpern, S. and Shocket, G. (1990) *Models of Clinical Management*. Institute of Health Services Management, London.

Donaldson, P. and Farquhar, J. (1988) *Understanding the British Economy*. Penguin, London.

Dowie, J. and Elstein, A. (eds) (1988) *Professional Judgement: A Reader in Clinical Decisionmaking*. Cambridge University Press, Cambridge.

Drucker, P. (1955) *The Practice of Management*. Pan Books, London.

Drucker, P. (1982) *The Age of Discontinuity*. HarperCollins, New York.

Dunleavy, P. (1989) 'The architecture of the British central state: Part 1: framework for analysis', *Public Administration*, 67(3): 249–76.

Dunleavy, P. (1991) *Democracy, Bureaucracy and Public Choice: Economic Explanations in Political Science*. Harvester Wheatsheaf, London.

Dunsire, A. (1978) *Implementation in a Bureaucracy: The Executive Process Part I*. Martin Robertson and Oxford University Press, London.

Enthoven, A.C. (1978) 'Consumer-choice health plan: inflation and inequity in health care today: alternatives for cost control and an analysis of proposals for National Health Insurance', *New England Journal of Medicine*, 298: 650–58 and 709–20.

Enthoven, A.C. (1985a) *Reflections on the Management of the National Health Service: An American Looks at Incentives to Efficiency in Health Services Management in the UK*. Nuffield Provincial Hospitals Trust, London.

Enthoven, A.C. (1985b) 'National Health Service: some reforms that might be politically feasible', *The Economist*, 22 June.

Esland, G. (1980) 'Professions and professionalism'. In Esland, G. and Salaman, G. (eds) *The Politics of Work and Occupations*. Open University Press, Milton Keynes.

Etzioni, A. (ed.) (1969) *The Semi-Professions and their Organisation*. Free Press, New York.

Feldman, R., Chan, H.C., Kralewski, J. *et al.* (1990) 'Effects of HMOs on the creation of competitive markets for hospital services', *Journal of Health Economics*, 9: 207–22.

Fitzgerald, L. (1991a) 'Made to measure', *Health Service Journal*, 31 October, pp. 24–5.

Fitzgerald, L. (1991b) 'This year's model', *Health Service Journal*, 7 November, pp. 26–7.

Flynn, N. (1990) *Public Sector Management*. Harvester Wheatsheaf, Hemel Hempstead.

Flynn, R. (1988) *Cutback Management in Health Services*. University of Salford Department of Sociology and Anthropology, Salford.

Fox, A. (1966) *Industrial Sociology and Industrial Relations*. HMSO, London.

Frater, A. and Spiby, J. (1990) *Measures Progress: Audit for Physicians: A Manual of Theory and Practice*. North West Thames Regional Health Authority, London.

Glennerster, H., Matsaganis, M. and Owens, P. (1992) *A Foothold for Fundholding: A Preliminary Report on the Introduction of GP Fundholding*. King's Fund, London.

Grant, W. (1985) 'Introduction'. In Grant, W. (ed.) *The Political Economy of Corporatism*. Macmillan, London.

Green, A. and Harrison, S. (1989) 'Efficiency and perversity in hospital services', *Health Services Management*, 85(3): 134–6.

Griggs, E. (1991) 'The politics of health reform', *Political Quarterly*, 62(4): 419–30.

Gruer, R., Gordon, D.S., Gunn, A.A. and Ruckley, C.V. (1986) 'Audit of surgical audit', *Lancet*, 4 January, pp. 23–5.

Ham, C.J. (1992) *Locality Purchasing*, Discussion Paper 30. University of Birmingham Health Services Management Centre, Birmingham.

Ham, C.J. and Heginbotham, C. (1992) *Purchasing Dilemmas*. King's Fund, London.

Ham, C.J. and Hunter, D.J. (1988) *Managing Clinical Activity in the NHS*, Briefing Paper No. 8. King's Fund Institute, London.

Handy, C. (1976) *Understanding Organisations*. Penguin, Harmondsworth.

Handy, C. (1985) *The Future of Work: A Guide to a Changing Society*. Blackwell, Oxford.

Handy, C. (1989) *The Age of Unreason*. Arrow Books, London.

Harrison, M.L. (1984) 'Themes and objectives'. In Harrison, M.L. (ed.) *Corporatism and the Welfare State*. Gower, Aldershot.

Harrison, S. (1981) 'The politics of health manpower'. In Long, A.F. and Mercer, G. (eds) *Manpower Planning in the National Health Service*. Gower Press, Farnborough.

Harrison, S. (1982) 'Consensus decisionmaking in the National Health Service: a review', *Journal of Management Studies*, 19(4): 377–94.

Harrison, S. (1984) 'Did consensus fail?', *Senior Nurse*, 1(2), 11 April: 16–18.

Harrison, S. (1988) *Managing the National Health Service: Shifting the Frontier?* Chapman and Hall, London.

Harrison, S. (1989) 'Industrial relations at national level'. In Connah, B.

and Lancaster, S. (eds) *The National Health Service Handbook*, 4th edn, 194–96. Macmillan/National Association of Health Authorities in England and Wales, London.

Harrison, S. (1991) 'Working the markets: purchaser/provider separation in English health care', *International Journal of Health Services*, 21(4): 625–35.

Harrison, S. (1992) 'Management and doctors'. In Bhugra, D. and Burns, A. (eds) *Management Training for Psychiatrists*. Gaskell, London.

Harrison, S. and Wistow, G. (1992) 'The purchaser/provider split in English, health care: towards explicit rationing?', *Policy and Politics*, 20(2).

Harrison, S., Hunter, D.J. and Pollitt, C.J. (1990) *The Dynamics of British Health Policy*. Unwin Hyman, London.

Harrison, S., Hunter, D.J., Marnoch, G. and Pollitt, C.J. (1992) *Just Managing: Power and Culture in the National Health Service*. Macmillan, London.

Haywood S.C. and Alaszewski, A. (1980) *Crisis in the Health Service: The Politics of Management*. Croom Helm, London.

Heginbotham, C. (1992) 'Rationing', *British Medical Journal*, 304: 496–9.

Henderson, J., Goldacre, M.J., Graveney, M.J. and Simmons, H.M. (1989) 'Use of medical record linkage to study readmission rates', *British Medical Journal*, 295: 1105–8.

Henley, D., Holtham, C., Likierman, A. and Perrin, J.R. (1986) *Public Sector Accounting and Financial Control*. Van Nostrand Reinhold/CIPFA, Wokingham.

Heyssel, R.M., Gaintner, J.R., Kues, I.W. *et al.* (1984) 'Decentralised management in a teaching hospital', *New England Journal of Medicine*, 310(22): 1477–80.

H.M. Treasury (1991) *Competing for Quality: Buying Better Public Services*, Cm. 1730. HMSO, London.

Hodges, C. (1991) 'Metamorphosis in the NHS: the personnel implications of Trust status', *Personnel Management*, April: 44–7.

Hopkins, A. (1991) 'Approaches to medical audit', *Journal of Epidemiology and Community Health*, (45): 1–3.

Hornbrook, M.C. (1982) 'Hospital casemix: its definition, measurement and use', *Medical Care Review*, 39(1): 1–43 and 73–123.

Hornbrook, M.C. and Berki, S.E. (1985) 'Practice mode and payment method: effects on use, costs, quality and access', *Medical Care*, 23(5): 484–511.

Hunter, D.J. (1992) 'Doctors as managers: poachers turned gamekeepers?', *Social Science and Medicine*, 35(4): 557–66.

Institute of Health Services Management (1988) *Working Party on Alternative Delivery and Funding of Health Services: Final Report*. IHSM, London.

Jenkins, L., Bardsley, M., Coles, J. *et al.* (1987) *Use and Validity of NHS*

*Performance Indicators – A National Survey.* CASPE Research/King's Fund, London.

Jenkins-Clarke, S. and Carr-Hill, R. (1991) *Nursing Workload Measures and Case Mix: An Investigation of the Reliability and Validity of Nursing Workload Measures.* University of York Centre for Health Economics, York.

Johnson, T.J. (1972) *Professions and Power.* Macmillan, London.

Jones, G. (1992) 'Bothering to remove gag on NHS staff', *Daily Telegraph,* 12 June, p. 1.

Kanter, R.M. (1990) *When Giants Learn to Dance: Mastering the Challenges of Strategy, Management and Careers in the 1990s.* Unwin Hyman, London.

Keynes, J.M. (1936) *The General Theory of Employment, Interest and Money.* Macmillan, London.

King Edward's Hospital Fund for London (1967) *The Shape of Hospital Management in 1980?* KEHFL, London.

Kingdon, J.W. (1984) *Agendas, Alternatives and Public Policies.* Little, Brown, Boston.

Klein, R.E. (1983) *The Politics of the National Health Service.* Longman, London.

Klein, R.E. (1989) *The Politics of the National Health Service,* 2nd edn, 182. Longman, London.

Klein, R.E. (1992) 'Dilemmas and decisions', *Health Management Quarterly,* 14(2): 2–5.

Laing, W. (1992) *UK Specialists' Fees – Is the Price Right?* Norwich Union Healthcare, Eastleigh.

Larkin, G.V. (1983) *Occupational Monopoly and Modern Medicine.* Tavistock, London.

Leathard, A. (1990) *Health Care Provision: Past, Present and Future.* Chapman and Hall, London.

LeGrand, J. (1990) *Quasi-markets and social policy.* University of Bristol School for Advanced Urban Studies, Bristol.

Levacic, R. (1987) *Economic Policy Making: Its Theory and Practice.* Wheatsheaf, Brighton.

Levitt, R. and Wall, A. (1992) *The Reorganised National Health Service,* 4th edn. Chapman and Hall, London.

Likierman, A. (1988) *Public Expenditure: Who Really Controls It and How.* Penguin, Harmondsworth.

Limb, M. (1992) 'GP fundholders force hospitals to cut jobs and beds', *Health Service Journal,* 6 August: 7.

Lipsky, M. (1980) *Street-Level Bureaucracy.* Russell Sage Foundation, New York.

Lomas, J. (1991) 'Words without action? The production, dissemination and impact of consensus recommendations', *Annual Review of Public Health,* 12: 41–65.

Long, A.F. and Sheldon, T.A. (1992) 'Enhancing effective and acceptable purchasing and providing decisions: overview and methods', *Quality in Health Care*, 1: 74–6.

Lukes, S. (1974) *Power: A Radical View*. Macmillan, London.

Mailly, R., Dimmock, S.J. and Sethi, A.S. (eds) (1989) *Industrial Relations in the Public Services*. Routledge, London.

McKee, M. and Lessof, L. (1992) 'Nurse and doctor: whose task is it anyway?'. In Robinson, J., Gray, A. and Elkan, R. (eds) *Policy Issues in Nursing*. Open University Press, Buckingham.

Mullen, P.M. (1985) 'Performance Indicators – is anything new?', *Hospital and Health Services Review*, 81(4): 165–7.

National Audit Office (1985) *Report by the Comptroller and Auditor General: NHS: Control of Nursing Manpower*. HMSO, London.

National Audit Office (1986) *Report by the Comptroller and Auditor General: Value for Money Developments in the National Health Service*. HMSO, London.

National Audit Office (1988) *Quality of Clinical Care in National Health Service Hospitals*, HC 736. HMSO, London.

Niskanen, W.A. (1971) *Bureaucracy and Representative Government*. Aldine-Atherton, Chicago.

Niskanen, W.A. (1973) *Bureaucracy: Servant or Master? Lessons from America*. Institute for Economic Affairs, London.

O'Connor, J. (1973) *The Fiscal Crisis of the State*. St. Martin's Press, New York.

Offe, C. (1984) *Contradictions of the Welfare State* (edited and translated by J. Keane). Hutchinson, London.

O'Sullivan, J. (1992) 'NHS operations delayed by Charter', *The Guardian*, 5 March, p. 2.

Packwood, T. (1991) 'The three faces of medical audit', *Health Service Journal*, 26 September, 24–6.

Packwood, T., Keen, J. and Buxton, M. (1991) *Hospitals in Transition: The Resource Management Experiment*. Open University Press, Milton Keynes.

Packwood, T., Keen, J. and Buxton, M. (1992) 'Process and structure: resource management and the development of sub-unit organisational structure', *Health Services Management Research*, 5(1): 66–76.

Parkhouse, J., Ellin, D.J. and Parkhouse, H.F. (1988) 'The views of doctors on management and administration', *Community Medicine*, 10: 25.

Parry, N. and Parry, J. (1976) *The Rise of the Medical Profession*. Croom Helm, London.

Peck, E. (1991) 'Power in the National Health Service: a case study of a unit considering NHS Trust status', *Health Services Management Research*, 4(2): 120–30.

Perey, B.J. (1984) 'The role of the physician manager', *Health Forum*, 48–55.

Perrin, J. (1988) *Resource Management in the NHS*. Van Nostrand Reinhold, Wokingham.

Peters, T.J. and Waterman, R.H. (1982) *In Search of Excellence*. Harper and Row, New York.

Pfeffer, N. and Coote, A. (1991) *Is Quality Good for You? A Critical Review of Quality Assurance in Welfare Services*. Institute for Public Policy Research, London.

Pfeffer, J. and Salancik, G.R. (1978) *The External Control of Organisations: A Resource Dependence Perspective*. Harper and Row, New York.

Pinch, T., Mulkay, M. and Ashmore, M. (1989) 'Clinical budgeting: experimentation in the social sciences: a drama in five acts', *Accounting Organisations and Society*, 14(3): 271–301.

Pollitt, C.J. (1985a) 'Measuring performance: a new system for the National Health Service', *Policy and Politics*, 13(1): 1–15.

Pollitt, C.J. (1985b) 'Can practice be made perfect?', *Health and Social Service Journal*, 6 June: 706–7.

Pollitt, C.J. (1991) 'The emergence of public service management', Unit 1 of *B.887 Managing Public Services*. The Open University, Milton Keynes.

Pollitt, C.J. (1993) *Managerialism and the Public Services: Cuts or Cultural Change?*, 2nd edn. Blackwell, Oxford.

Pollitt, C.J., Harrison, S., Hunter, D.J. and Marnoch, G. (1988) 'The reluctant managers: clinicians and budgets in the NHS', *Financial Accountability and Management*, 4(3): 213–33.

Rhodes, R.A.W. (1986) 'Corporate bias in central–local relations: a case study of the consultative council on local government finance', *Policy and Politics*, 14(2): 221–45.

Robinson, K. (1992) 'The nursing workforce: aspects of "inequality"'. In Robinson, J., Gray, A. and Elkan, R. (eds) *Policy Issues in Nursing*. Open University Press, Buckingham.

Robinson, R. and Judge, K. (1987) *Public Expenditure and the NHS: Trends and Prospects*. King's Fund Institute, London.

Royal College of Nursing (1989) *A Framework for Quality: a Patient-centred Approach to Quality Assurance in Health Care*. Royal College of Nursing, London.

Royal College of Physicians (1989) *Medical Audit: A First Report: What, Why and How?* Royal College of Physicians, London.

Royal College of Surgeons of London (1990) *Report of the National CEPOD 1989*. RCS, London.

Russell, I.T., Addington-Hall, J.M., Avery, P.J. *et al.* (1992) 'Medical audit in general practice II: effects on health of patients with common childhood conditions', *British Medical Journal*, 304: 1484–8.

Sale, D. (1990) *Essentials of Nursing Management: Quality Assurance*. Macmillan, Baskingstoke.

Saltman, R.B. and von Otter, C. (1987) 'Re-vitalising public health care systems: a proposal for public competition in Sweden', *Health Policy*, 7(1): 21–40.

Saltman, R.B. and von Otter, C. (1989) 'Public competition versus mixed markets: an analytic comparison', *Health Policy*, 11(1): 43–55.

Saltman, R.B. and von Otter, C. (1990) 'Implementing public competition in Swedish county councils: a case study', *International Journal of Health Planning and Management*, 5(2): 105–16.

Saltman, R.B. and von Otter, C. (1992) *Planned Markets and Public Competition: Strategic Reform in Northern European Health Systems.* Open University Press, Buckingham.

Saltman R.B., Harrison S. and von Otter, C. (1990) 'Competition and public funds'. In Paine, L.H.W. (ed.) *National Association of Health Care Supplies Managers Members' Reference Book and Buyers' Guide*, 64–66. Sterling, London.

Salvage, J. (1992) 'The new nursing: empowering patients or empowering nurses?'. In Robinson, J., Gray, A. and Elkan, R. (eds) *Policy Issues in Nursing.* Open University Press, Buckingham.

Schmitter, P.C. (1974) 'Still the century of corporatism?', *Review of Politics*, 36: 85–131.

Schulz, R.I. and Harrison, S. (1986) 'Physician autonomy in the Federal Republic of Germany, Great Britain, and the United States, *International Journal of Health Planning and Management*, 1(5): 335–55.

Schulz, R.I. and Johnson, A.C. (1990) *Management of Hospitals and Health Services*, 3rd edn. C.V. Mosby, St. Louis.

Scrivens, E. (1988) 'The management of clinicians in the National Health Service', *Social Policy and Administration*, 22(1): 22–34.

Seifert, R. (1992) *Industrial Relations in the NHS.* Chapman and Hall, London.

Smith, I.J. (1992) 'Ethics and health care rationing – new challenges for the public sector manager', *Journal of Management in Medicine*, 6(1): 54–61.

Smith, N. and Chantler, C. (1987) 'Partnership for progress', *Public Finance and Accountancy*, pp. 12–14.

Smith, R., Grabham, A. and Chantler, C. (1989) 'Doctors becoming managers', *British Medical Journal*, 298: 311.

Starkey, K. (1992) 'Time and the consultant: issues of contract and control'. In Loveridge, R. and Starkey, K. (eds) *Continuity and Crisis in the NHS.* Open University Press, Buckingham.

Stewart, J. (1990) 'Local government: new thinking on neglected issues', *Public Money and Management*, 10(2): 59–60.

Stewart, R., Gabbay, J., Dopson, S. *et al.* (1987) *Managing with Doctors: Working Together?*, Issue Study No. 5. Templeton College, Oxford.

Stocking, B. (1985) *Initiative and Inertia: Case Studies in the NHS.* Nuffield Provincial Hospitals Trust, London.

Stocking, B. (1992) 'Promoting change in clinical care', *Quality in Health Care*, 1: 56–60.

Symes, D. (1992) 'Resource management in the National Health Service'. In Pollitt, C.J. and Harrison, S. (eds) *Handbook of Public Service Management*. Blackwell, Oxford.

Taylor-Gooby, P. (1985) 'The politics of welfare: public attitudes and behaviour'. In Klein, R.E. and O'Higgins, M. (eds) *The Future of Welfare*. Blackwell, Oxford.

Taylor-Gooby, P. (1987) 'Citizenship and welfare'. In Jowell, R., Witherspoon, S. and Brook, L. (eds) *British Social Attitudes: the 1987 Report*. Gower, Aldershot.

Thain C. and Wright, M. (1991) 'Trends in public expenditure', *B887: Managing Public Services*, Unit 3. Open University, Milton Keynes.

Tolliday, H. (1978) 'Clinical autonomy'. In Jacques, E. (ed.) *Health Services: Their Nature and Organisation and the Role of Patients, Doctors, and the Health Professions*. Heinemann, London.

Tomlin, Z. (1992) 'Their treatment in your hands', *The Guardian*, 29 April, p. 21.

Tomlin, Z. (1993) 'New Trust contract rules out "moonlighting" by consultants', *Health Service Journal*, 18 February, p. 4.

Vickers, G. (1965) *The Art of Judgement*. Chapman and Hall, London.

Viefhues, H. (ed.) (1988) *Medical Manpower in the European Community*. Springer-Verlag, Berlin.

Ware, J.E., Brook, R.H., Rogers, W.R. *et al.* (1986) 'Comparison of health outcomes at a health maintenance organisation with those of fee-for-service care', *The Lancet*, 3 May, pp. 107–22.

Watkin, B. (1975) *Documents on Health and Social Services: 1834 to the Present Day*. Methuen, London.

Watkin, B. (1978) *The National Health Service: The First Phase – 1948–1974 and After*. Allen and Unwin, London.

Weiner, J.P. and Ferriss, D.M. (1990) *GP Budget Holding in the UK: Lessons from America*, Research Report No. 7. King's Fund Institute, London.

Wickings, I. (1983) 'Consultants face the figures', *Health and Social Service Journal*, 8 December, 1466–8.

Wickings, I., Coles, J., Flux, R. and Howard, L. (1983) 'Review of clinical budgeting and costing experiments', *British Medical Journal*, 286: 578.

Williamson, C. (1992) *Whose Standards? Consumer and Professional Standards in Health Care*. Open University Press, Buckingham.

World Health Organization (1989) *The Leningrad Experiment in Health Care Management*. World Health Organization Regional Office for Europe, Copenhagen.

Yates, J. (1983) 'When will the players get involved?', *Health and Social Service Journal*, 15 September: 1111–12.

Young, A. (1986) *Practical Management Budgeting in the NHS: A New Initiative for Successful Implementation*. Arthur Young, Glasgow.
Young, K. (1977) 'Values in the policy process', *Policy and Politics*, 5: 1–22.

# INDEX

**FINANCING HEALTH CARE IN THE 1990s**

**John Appleby**

The British National Health Service has embarked on a massive programme of change in the way it provides health care. The financing of the
Health Service is at the heart of this change and controversies over this issue
are likely to stay with us in the coming decade, whichever political party is
in power. This book explores some of the directions that the financing of
health care could take over the next ten years. For instance, will the
Conservative Government's stated commitment to a health care system
financed out of general taxation remain? Or, if the current reforms fail to
bring measurable benefits of any significance, will the political pressures to
take reforms even further lead to still greater changes in funding, financing
and operations? Will the state of the national economy necessitate further
reforms? Or might the reforms to date take an uncharted path with some
unexpected outcomes?

For the senior student, academic or health care professional this book
offers an expert's view of the financing of the Health Service now and in the
future.

### Contents
*New directions – Seeds of change – Past trends in health-care funding – The
right level of funding – A market for health care – Managing the market: the
US experience – Managing the market: the West German experience – Some
views of the future – Conclusions – References – Index.*

192pp      0 335 09776 6 (Paperback)      0 335 09777 4 (Hardback)

**PATIENTS, POLICIES AND POLITICS**
BEFORE AND AFTER *WORKING FOR PATIENTS*

**John Butler**

The 1989 White Paper *Working for Patients* was the watershed of the Conservative government's policymaking for the future of the British National Health Service. This book examines the political and historical background to the White Paper, its contents and proposals, and the actions and reactions to which it gave rise. The book is written in an accessible and jargon-free style and is aimed at a wide range of readers from various professional and academic backgrounds who are seeking a synoptic and balanced view of this remarkable episode in the history of the NHS.

*Contents*
*Origins – Context – Content – Purposes – Dissent – Prophecies – Implementation – Reflections – References – Index.*

160pp      0 335 15647 9 (Paperback)      0 335 15648 7 (Hardback)

## PUBLIC LAW AND HEALTH SERVICE ACCOUNTABILITY
**Diane Longley**

This book examines the relationship between the processes of accountability and management within the health service in the light of the recent
National Health Service and Community Care Act. The author argues that
health care is a social entitlement, to be moulded and allocated according to
rational social choices and to be protected from becoming a commodity
which is largely controlled by unaccountable market forces. Insufficient
attention has been given to the potential role of law in the shaping of health
policy and the management of the health service as a public organization.
The arguments put forward here rest on a firm belief in a constitutional
backcloth for the operation of all government and public services. The
author calls for greater openness in health policy planning, in management
and professional activities, the introduction of standards of conduct in
health service management and for the establishment of an independent
'Institute of Health' to analyse and advise on health policy.

This important and timely book will be of interest to a wide range of
students, academics and professionals interested in health service policy,
politics and management.

### Contents
*Diagnostic deficiencies: health policy, public law and public management –
Prescriptive dilemmas: accountability and the statutory and administrative
structure of the NHS – Cuts, sutures and costs: implementing policy and
monitoring standards – Patients and perseverance: grievances and resolution
– Sovereign remedies and preventive medicine: patient choice and markets –
Prognosis and preventive medicine: antidotes, tonics and learning –
Bibliography – Index.*

136pp     0 335 09685 9 (Paperback)     0 335 09686 7 (Hardback)

**HOSPITALS IN TRANSITION**
THE RESOURCE MANAGEMENT EXPERIMENT

**Tim Packwood, Justin Keen and Martin Buxton**

This book is the result of an evaluation commissioned by the Department of
Health, that has given the authors exceptional 'access to the six acute
hospital sites selected to pilot Resource Management (RM), over a three
year period. Introduced in these National Health hospitals in 1986, RM is
currently being implemented in all major hospitals. It was expected that
patient care would benefit from better management of resources: management that involved the service providers and was based upon data that
accurately recorded and costed their activities. This represented an
enormous cultural change moving away from the traditional hierarchical
and functional patterns of management.

The book draws upon close observation of the way in which RM has
developed both locally and nationally, supported by interviews with the
main participants, scrutiny of the documentation and specially designed
surveys. It will provide an invaluable introduction to RM for all health
service practitioners involved in management and to academics in health
studies and public administration.

***Contents***
*Introduction – RM in context – Project planning and management – The*
*implementation of RM – The RM process – The resource requirements of*
*RM – Benefits of RM – Conclusions and implications – The organization*
*transformed – Appendices – Glossary – References.*

208pp      0 335 09950 5 (Paperback)      0 335 09951 0 3 (Hardback)